HowExpert Guide to Diet and Nutrition

101 Tips to Learn about Diet and Nutrition, Eating the Right Foods for Essential Nutrients, and Becoming a Healthier Person

HowExpert with Lacy Ngo

For more tips related to this topic, visit HowExpert.com/dietnutrition.

Recommended Resources

- HowExpert.com – Quick 'How To' Guides on All Topics from A to Z by Everyday Experts.
- HowExpert.com/free – Free HowExpert Email Newsletter.
- HowExpert.com/books – HowExpert Books
- HowExpert.com/courses – HowExpert Courses
- HowExpert.com/clothing – HowExpert Clothing
- HowExpert.com/membership – HowExpert Membership Site
- HowExpert.com/affiliates – HowExpert Affiliate Program
- HowExpert.com/jobs – HowExpert Jobs
- HowExpert.com/writers – Write About Your #1 Passion/Knowledge/Expertise & Become a HowExpert Author.
- HowExpert.com/resources – Additional HowExpert Recommended Resources
- YouTube.com/HowExpert – Subscribe to HowExpert YouTube.
- Instagram.com/HowExpert – Follow HowExpert on Instagram.
- Facebook.com/HowExpert – Follow HowExpert on Facebook.
- TikTok.com/@HowExpert – Follow HowExpert on TikTok.

Publisher's Foreword

Dear HowExpert Reader,

HowExpert publishes quick 'how to' guides on all topics from A to Z by everyday experts.

At HowExpert, our mission is to discover, empower, and maximize everyday people's talents to ultimately make a positive impact in the world for all topics from A to Z...one everyday expert at a time!

All of our HowExpert guides are written by everyday people just like you and me, who have a passion, knowledge, and expertise for a specific topic.

We take great pride in selecting everyday experts who have a passion, real-life experience in a topic, and excellent writing skills to teach you about the topic you are also passionate about and eager to learn.

We hope you get a lot of value from our HowExpert guides, and it can make a positive impact on your life in some way. All of our readers, including you, help us continue living our mission of positively impacting the world for all spheres of influences from A to Z.

If you enjoyed one of our HowExpert guides, then please take a moment to send us your feedback from wherever you got this book.

Thank you, and we wish you all the best in all aspects of life.

Sincerely,

BJ Min
Founder & Publisher of HowExpert
HowExpert.com

PS...If you are also interested in becoming a HowExpert author, then please visit our website at HowExpert.com/writers. Thank you & again, all the best!

Table of Contents

Chapter 1: Where to Look to Learn about Diet and Nutrition?

We are bombarded with tips, fad diets, pills, and supplements that claim to be the key to optimal health and well-being. With all this information, how do we know what is true? This book is going to break down the nutrition basics for you.

In this book, you will learn:

- What a healthy diet actually looks like?
- What nutrients should you focus on eating and why?
- What supplements work, based on research?
- Where should you look to get accurate nutrition information?

First, let's focus on the last bullet.

Where should you look to get accurate nutrition information?

This is probably the first step to eating healthier. If you don't know where to get your nutrition information, you will just be spinning in circles trying to figure out what you should actually be doing.

When you are reading nutrition information on websites, look to see who is writing it. If the nutrition article is written by a registered dietitian, then you are off to a great start on your health journey

Tip 1: Look for an RD or RDN beside someone's name. Dietitians have extensive nutrition education and knowledge.

Registered dietitians require extensive nutrition education to become licensed and are considered THE experts in human nutrition. They are more trained in the nutrition field than most doctors, personal trainers, and nutritionists (in the US). A nutritionist in the United States may or may not have nutrition education because the term nutritionist is not regulated. In other words, anyone can legally call themselves a nutritionist.

Doctors usually have some knowledge in nutrition but often not as much nutrition knowledge as a dietitian. On the other hand, doctors are vastly knowledgeable in other areas but often only take one nutrition course throughout their education.

Personal trainers are knowledgeable in physical fitness and exercise but will usually only have general nutrition knowledge.

On the other hand, becoming a registered dietitian usually takes about five to six years of higher education and an internship. Registered Dietitians are required to complete a bachelor's degree at a college accredited by the Commission of Accreditation of Dietetic Education. The required classes generally include Medical Nutrition Therapy, Microbiology, Biology, Organic Chemistry, Anatomy and physiology, Evidence-Based Nutrition, Human Nutrition and Metabolism, and Nutrition Counseling, to name a few courses.

After they have acquired their bachelor's degree in human nutrition, they still don't have enough to become a licensed dietitian yet. Next, they must complete 1200 hours of a competitive internship program.

After they have obtained their bachelor's degree and completed the internship program; then they must take the grueling CDR exam, and by the year 2024, registered dietitians will be required to have a master's degree as well.

Dietitians are also required to stay up to date by completing continuing education units throughout their careers.

So, you can see why dietitians are a good start when looking for someone who understands the science of nutrition. However, that does not mean that nutritionists and health coaches do not bring value to the nutrition conversation. Many have done their research and are very knowledgeable, and some health coaches and nutritionists have some formal training or some type of certifications, but not always.

Tip 2: If the person sharing nutrition information is not a dietitian, they may still be knowledgeable. Look to see where they get their information. Do they get the information from a dietitian?

When you do find information written by health coaches, nutritionists, or health enthusiasts, look to see where they are getting their information. Do they quote dietitians? Then, they may be getting their information from a reliable source. People who are passionate about their transformation journey can also write informative and inspiring information, but after you read their stories, you should verify their information through a dietitian.

Tip 3: If you have been inspired by someone's health transformation story, verify their information by researching what a dietitian says about their strategy.

Dietitians are not all equally knowledgeable, but when you see an RD or RDN by someone's name, at the very least, you know they had years of extensive nutrition education.

Think of Me as Your Dietitian Resource Throughout This Book

While you are reading this book, you can think of me as your dietitian resource. As your dietitian resource, I am going to try to answer all of your basic nutrition questions.

Here is a little background about your dietitian resource (aka me):

I am a registered dietitian with a Bachelor's of Science in Human Nutrition from Clemson University and a Master's of Science from Winthrop University. I taught nutrition at Winthrop University as well.

But there is more to my story. I have not only a professional nutrition background but also a personal transformation story.

I am a registered dietitian who lost 50 pounds after I transformed my way of eating, and this transformation happened after I stopped focusing on my weight and started focusing on my health.

*Below are before and after my health transformation pictures.

Before

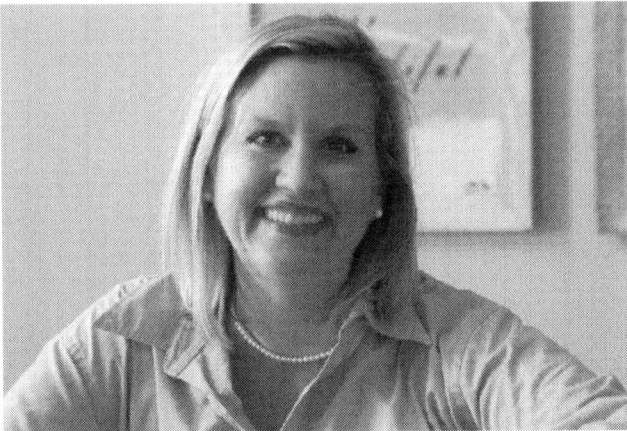

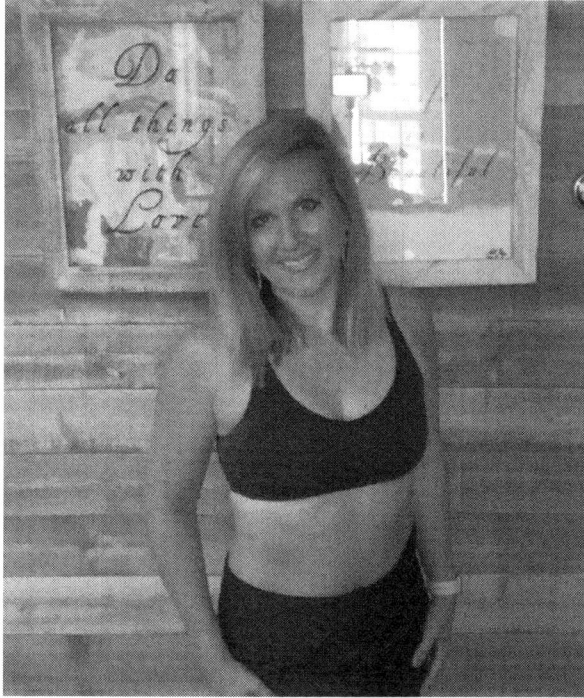

After

I decided to make this change when I noticed I was feeling sad more often than usual. I was also getting sick more frequently, and my seasonal allergies were becoming more and more severe. In addition, I was experiencing hip pain and feelings of brain fog, and lack of energy. Brain fog is when you feel like you are not as alert or quick thinking as you would like to be. With brain fog, you feel like you are not fully aware of your surroundings and have trouble staying focused.

The amazing point of this story is that when I started focusing on eating the foods that helped my body, brain, and mood, all my symptoms significantly (and I mean significantly) improved.

My mood improved, and I had more energy. I rarely get sick now, and my allergies and hip pain have almost disappeared. I am now more alert, focused, and relaxed. And as a bonus, I even lost 50 pounds.

So, I understand what science says about nutrition, and I can personally attest to the impact food can have on our health.

Throughout this book, I want to share what nutrients your mind and body need for optimal health.

Review of Chapter 1

- Registered dietitians have years of extensive education and are usually one of the best resources for nutrition information.
- Think of me as your dietitian resource during this book.
- Nutrition can have an impact on our mind, body, and mood.
- Throughout this book, I am going to share my nutrition knowledge based on my education and personal story.

*Below are a few more before and after transformation pictures.

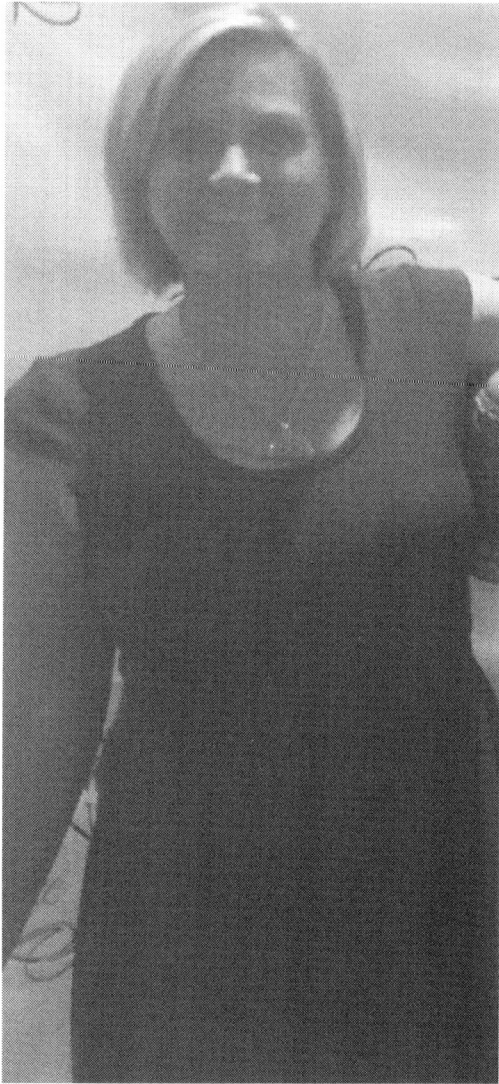

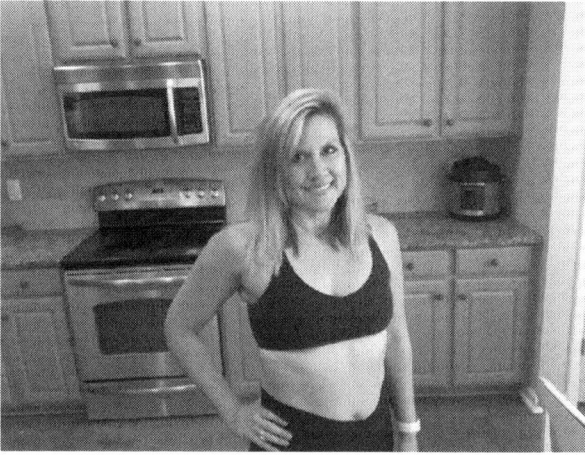

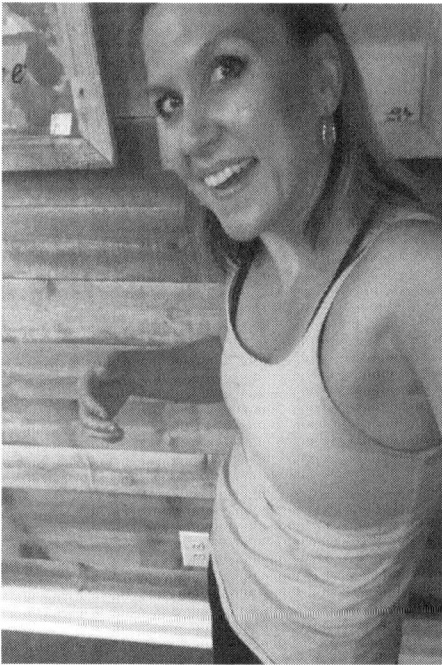

Chapter 2: The "Right" Foods and Essential Nutrients for the Mind

A healthy diet provides nutrients that will help the whole person-mind and body. When we are eating foods for the mind, we are eating foods that help with mood and reduce the risk or decrease the symptoms of mood disorders, like depression, anxiety, and feelings of stress. Our moods and energy levels can affect our behaviors and actions. We sometimes make poor decisions when we act without thinking, lose our temper often, or make small things into big things. These decisions affect our relationships and our outlook on life, which leads to a poor mood. And now we have come full circle. Our poor moods and lack of energy affect our actions, and our actions affect our mood.

When we are eating foods for the mind, we are also eating foods that may help with memory and brain function and reduce the risk of cognitive decline, dementia, and Alzheimer's as we age.

Food and Mood

This topic is near and dear to me because my mood transformed when I became intentional about eating mood-boosting foods. For this section, I have made a list of nutrients that impact our mood and mood disorders based on research. So, let's dive into the nutrient research.

Antioxidants and Mood

First up... antioxidants.

If you decide you can only change one aspect of your diet, then you may want it to be this: Eat more foods with antioxidants.

Antioxidants are, dare I say, magical? No really, it's not magic... it's science, but the impact they have on our health may feel like magic. To put it simply, antioxidants are a substance that stops oxidation. Oxidation increases free radicals in the body, and antioxidants get rid of free radicals in the body. Unfortunately, these free radicals cause a multitude of problems, including increased signs of aging, reduced brain function, and an increased risk of chronic diseases, cancer, and chronic inflammation. Chronic inflammation also increases the risk of chronic diseases and stress, and depression (12, 57).

There are a vast number of different types of antioxidants. Some are more beneficial than others, and different antioxidants appear helpful in different parts of the body. This is why eating an array of antioxidant-containing foods is important. Beneficial antioxidants include, but are not limited to, polyphenols like flavonoid quercetin, beta-carotene (Vitamin A), Vitamin E, Vitamin C, Selenium, zinc, selenium, lutein, zeaxanthin, catechins, resveratrol, Sulforaphane, and anthocyanin flavonoid. In addition, antioxidants are found in fruits, vegetables, nuts, seeds, tea, olive oil, whole grains, dark chocolate, and herbs and spices like sage, rosemary, and garlic.

Tip 4: Eat more fruits, vegetables, nuts, seeds, tea, olive oil, whole grains, and dark chocolate to get more antioxidants in your diet.

According to two meta-analyses, diets high in these antioxidant-rich foods were associated with a decreased risk of depression (68, 110). Inversely, studies, including a meta-analysis that looked at ten studies, found that people with depression tend to have lower antioxidant intakes (11, 31, 100). Another study found that when individuals drank four or more cups of antioxidant-containing green tea, they had a 51% lower prevalence of depression compared to individuals who drank one cup or less per day, which contains flavanol polyphenol antioxidants. Polyphenol flavonoids are the powerful antioxidants you find in green tea (104).

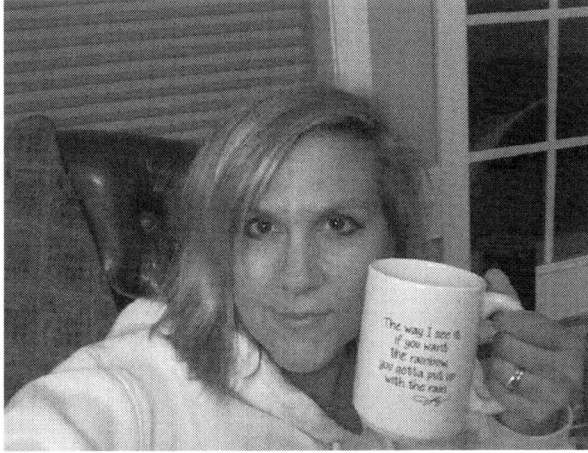

In another study, if participants were given Vitamin C supplements just before a stressful task, their cortisol stress hormone levels returned to normal more quickly, indicating that vitamin C may play a role in stress management. In addition, vitamin C has powerful antioxidant properties (31).

Tip 5: To satisfy your sweet tooth, eat one small piece of decadent dark chocolate.

Dark chocolate is so strong that you don't need much to satisfy your craving. Plus, dark chocolate contains flavonoid antioxidants.

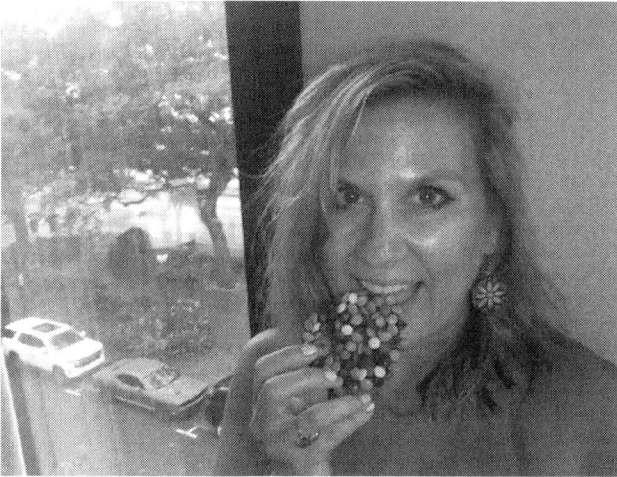

Omega-3 and Mood

Omega-3 is an anti-inflammatory nutrient, and according to ample research, Omega-3 is another important nutrient when it comes to mood. In addition, Omega-3 may have a calming effect because it helps regulate neurotransmitters (122). In fact, in some studies, Omega-3 supplements appeared as effective as anti-depressant medications for some individuals (11).

Fish like salmon and tuna are fantastic sources of Omega-3. One review of 31 studies found that fish consumption decreased depression symptoms. Another study found that people who ate salmon three times a week for five months reported less anxiety (37).

Omega-3 seems to have a positive effect on anxiety symptoms as well. In a double-blinded randomized study, omega-3 supplements appeared to help with anxiety levels of young athletes when they were faced with a stressful exam (122).

Salmon, tuna, walnuts, chia seeds, flaxseeds, and hemp seeds are all excellent sources of Omega-3. Tuna and salmon not only contain omega-3 but are also good sources of selenium. Selenium is a mineral with antioxidant properties. Salmon and tuna contain vitamin D as well. As you will read later, vitamin D plays an important role when it comes to our mood.

Tip 7: Include antioxidant and ALA omega-3-rich nuts and seeds in your diet.

Walnuts, chia seeds, flaxseeds, and hemp seeds are rich in antioxidants and plant-based Omega-3s.

B Vitamins and Mood

Ample studies have shown that low vitamin B levels, especially vitamin B12 and folate levels, are associated with an increased risk of depression. In fact, severe vitamin B12 deficiencies can double the risk of severe depression (11). Nourishing foods that contain B vitamins include lean meats, salmon, dairy, eggs, legumes, dark leafy vegetables, and whole grains.

Tip 8: Include nourishing foods like lean meats, salmon, dairy, eggs, legumes, dark leafy green vegetables, or whole grains in your diet.

Vitamin B levels tend to decrease with age; therefore, some older adults may need B vitamin supplements as well. Check your levels with your doctor before adding a supplement.

Vitamin D, Zinc, Riboflavin, and Magnesium and Mood

According to research, deficiencies in any one of these nutrients (vitamin D, zinc, riboflavin, and magnesium) are associated with an increased risk of depression and anxiety (9, 39, 65, 96). For example, according to one study, vitamin D deficiency is associated with an 8-14% increased risk of depression (119).

Tip 9: To get adequate vitamin D, go outside and enjoy the sun, but remember to wear sunscreen.

You can get vitamin D from salmon, tuna, and cage-free eggs; however, one of the best sources of vitamin D is sunlight.

Magnesium is found in foods like whole grains, nuts, seeds, avocados, and dark chocolate.

Animal proteins are a good source of zinc, but you can also find zinc in nuts, seeds, legumes, oats, and tofu.

Probiotics and Mood

It has been well established that gut health plays a significant role in our mood. Probiotics, which are good bacteria for our bodies, are important for gut health, and several studies and systemic reviews, including double-blinded placebo-controlled studies, have indicated that probiotics, specifically, may reduce symptoms of anxiety, depression, and stress (4, 11, 48, 83, 108, 123).

The gut may play a role in our mood because the gut and brain are directly connected by way of the vagus nerve. The vagus nerve can send messages from the gut to the brain and vice versa. This connection is called the gut-brain axis. Moreover, 95% of serotonin, which regulates mood, is found in the GI tract. Ninety-five percent of serotonin, the neurotransmitter that helps regulate mood, sleep, appetite, and pain, is found in the gut (129). Probiotic sources include yogurt, kimchi, fermented sour kraut, fermented pickles, kombucha, and kefir.

Tip 10: Try eating yogurt, berries, and nuts for breakfast.

This breakfast is packed with probiotics, fiber, protein, and antioxidants!

Fiber and Mood

We can't talk about gut health without mentioning fiber. Prebiotic fiber feeds probiotics. And just like probiotics, Studies have found a link between diets low in fiber and prebiotic fiber and depression and anxiety (80). Fiber also helps you feel full, which can help with weight loss when needed.

Tip 11: Include fiber at every meal to support gut health and help with portion control.

Good sources of fiber include fruits, vegetables, whole grains, beans, nuts, and seeds.

A Note on Tart Cherries

Tip 12: If you are having trouble sleeping, try drinking some light cherry juice before bed.

It is well-known that lack of sleep increases feelings of depression, anxiety, and stress. Melatonin is a substance in the body that helps us fall asleep and stay asleep. Tart cherries are one of the few foods that contain natural melatonin, and according to a study published in the European Journal of Nutrition, tart cherry juice may improve sleep (45).

Hydration and Mood

Tip 13: Fill up a large water bottle with water first thing in the morning. Keep the water bottle with you and take sips of water throughout the day to stay hydrated.

Drinking water throughout the day is critical for your body and your mood. In fact, dehydration can cause significant negative changes in mood and promote feelings of restlessness (11).

Tip 14: If you don't love the taste of water, try adding lemon or fruit to your water to add flavor..

Foods that Could Have a Negative Impact on Your Mood

Studies, including a study that looked at 8,964 participants, have found a link between diets high in sugar, trans fat, energy-dense/low-nutrient foods, and ultra-processed foods, like commercially baked goods and depression and anxiety. Another study found an increase in depression scores among children who consumed sugary soft drinks. In addition, these foods are pro-inflammatory, increase oxidative stress, and disturb the gut microbiome balance (11, 32).

Tip 15: Only occasionally eat inflammatory foods that increase your risk of depression, anxiety, and stress.

These foods include high sugar foods like commercially baked goods, trans fat foods, ultra-processed foods, and energy-dense, low nutrient foods..

Food Sensitivity and Mood

If you are sensitive or allergic to certain foods, then eating these foods could negatively affect your mood (1). The most common food sensitivities and intolerances are gluten, dairy, soy, yeast, corn, eggs, nuts, histamine, FODMAPS, nightshade vegetables, cruciferous vegetables. However, as you can see, some of these foods are also full of extremely beneficial nutrients, so we only want to eliminate a food if you discover you are sensitive to it.

Tip 16: If you are sensitive or allergic to a food, eliminate that food from your diet.

If you are only sensitive and not allergic or intolerant to a food, you can sometimes add that food back into your diet after you have given your gut time to rest and heal.

Check with your doctor or dietitian before you eliminate foods.

You can become sensitive to food if you are eating a certain food too often. If this is the case, you can sometimes eliminate the food for 6 to 8 weeks and then add the food back into your diet. (Some people, however, will have to continue to eliminate permanently).

Tip 17: Eat a variety of grains throughout the day instead of just one type of grain.

Gluten is becoming a more common food sensitivity. If you think about it, gluten-containing wheat is one of the most common grains we eat in America. For example, it is not unusual for someone to eat pancakes for breakfast, a sandwich for lunch, and pizza for dinner. All of these contain either refined wheat or whole wheat. Both of which contain gluten. If we eat a variety of grains instead of just wheat, then we may be less likely to become sensitive to gluten. Whole grains include whole wheat, oats, quinoa, brown rice, and buckwheat (not wheat). Eating a variety of these foods will reduce the amount of gluten we are eating on a daily basis.

For example, one day, you may want to eat oatmeal for breakfast, a whole grain sandwich for lunch (contains gluten), and brown rice for dinner. Note, if you are already gluten sensitive, gluten intolerant, or have celiac disease, do not eat gluten.

Food and Brain Health: How Food Affects How Well We Think and Remember

Did you know that the foods we eat can impact our memory, ability to think quickly, test scores, and risk of Alzheimer's, dementia, and age-related cognitive decline (13, 43, 75, 86, 93)?

According to the research, the best diets for the brain are plant-based diets high in vegetables, fruits, nuts, seeds, legumes, whole grains, and moderate in cold-water fish. In addition, berries, leafy greens, and salmon have a significant positive impact on our brain's ability to function optimally (85).

Diets rich in vegetables, fruits, nuts, seeds, legumes, and whole grains are not only associated with a reduced risk of mood disorders but are also associated with a reduced risk of cognitive decline. In addition, these foods are also associated with better test scores, memory, and attention. For instance, in one study, researchers found that children who ate a breakfast consisting of whole grains vs. students who drank fruit juice for breakfast had higher scores in math and reading (105).

In another study, children who consumed a drink that contained a combination of vitamins and minerals and omega-3 scored higher on memory and verbal intelligence (32).

Inversely, diets high in trans-fat, saturated fat, salt, sugar, and ultra-processed foods are associated with a decline in brain function. In addition, foods that ranked higher on the glycemic index, i.e., refined carbohydrates and sugar, are associated with a negative impact on brain function, attention, and memory (74).

Tip 18: Limit sugary drinks and sodas.

Sugary drinks and sodas are low on nutrients and high on sugar and empty calories. (Side note, I had a client who lost 20 pounds by omitting sugary drinks from her diet. She didn't change anything else in her diet).

Tip 19: Only eat ultra-processed foods and foods that contain trans-fat, refined sugar, refined carbohydrates, salt, and saturated fat occasionally to promote optimal brain function.

So, we have established that food can significantly affect how well our brain functions, but what does the research say about individual nutrients??

Omega-3 and Brain Health

First, let's look at the nutrient that is known as the brain nutrient-Omega-3. Human and mice trials suggest that omega-3 may help prevent cognitive decline, reduce the risk of Alzheimer's and dementia in older adults, and improve school performance scores in children (32, 74, 93). After healthy older women were given DHA Omega-3 and lutein supplements for four months, their memory scores, verbal fluency, and rate of learning significantly improved (52).

A few human and mice studies even suggest that Omega-3 may positively impact brain function in individuals who have suffered a traumatic brain injury (41).

Probiotics and Brain Health

Remember those probiotics we discussed earlier? You know, that good bacteria in your gut that may offer protection against mood disorders? Well, those probiotics may also help with brain function as well.

Human and rat studies, including a double-blinded control trial, support the theory that probiotics promote brain function, focus, memory, and attention and may reduce the risk and/or slow the progression of Alzheimer's and dementia (2, 23, 26, 132). For example, in one study, when researchers gave lead-exposed rats probiotics, the rats' memory was repaired (132).

Tip 20: Aim to eat a probiotic-rich food 4 to 5 times a week.

Remember, probiotic-rich foods include yogurt, kefir, kombucha, miso, sour kraut, fermented pickles, and kimchi.

Antioxidants and Brain Health

Research suggests high antioxidant consumption through food is linked to improved brain function and reduced risk of Alzheimer's Disease and Dementia (6, 27). For example, one 3-year study showed lower intakes of vegetables and legumes, rich in antioxidants, were linked with cognitive decline in aging (21). Another study with a large sample size of 4,740 individuals 65 years old or older found that vitamin C and vitamin E supplementation reduced the prevalence of Alzheimer's by 78% (133). Yet another study found that increased serum levels of beta-carotene (an antioxidant) were linked to an 85% reduction in the risk of cognitive decline in older adults (46).

Tip 22: Try to eat a dark leafy green every day.

Kale, broccoli, strawberries, oranges, papayas, kiwi, Brussel Sprouts, dark leafy greens, and red, yellow, and green peppers are good sources of vitamin C.

Nuts, seeds, dark leafy greens, and broccoli contain Vitamin E.

Good sources of Beta-carotene are orange vegetables like pumpkin, sweet potatoes, and butternut squash, as well as dark leafy greens and broccoli.

Did you notice dark leafy greens are listed as a good source of vitamin E, vitamin C, and beta-carotene?

Tip 23: Eat berries at least two times a week.

Berries are rich in the antioxidants- anthocyanin and resveratrol. These antioxidants appear to offer significant protection from brain function decline.

Tip 23: Add berries to your cereal or yogurt for breakfast, or eat a handful of berries for a snack to make sure you are getting adequate berries into your diet.

In a randomized, double-blinded placebo-controlled study, older adults ate one cup of blueberries every day. They found that the participant's memory and ability to accurately switch tasks improved significantly after only 90 days (53, 81).

Tip 24: Add fresh herbs and spices to your recipes as much as possible.

Many spices and herbs are also rich in antioxidants. Turmeric is on spice that contains antioxidants. Scientists have noted that the prevalence of Alzheimer's is low in India, where turmeric consumption is high. Turmeric's positive impact on cognitive function has also been observed in animal studies: turmeric reduced memory and cognitive decline in animals with Alzheimer's or brain trauma (32).

Rosemary and Sage are two other flavorful spices that may protect the brain against cognitive decline. In a double-blinded, placebo-controlled study, rosemary significantly increased memory speed in older adults (6, 36, 101). Another double-blinded randomized, placebo-controlled study found that individuals with Alzheimer's disease who consumed common sage scored higher on memory, problem-solving, and reasoning tests compared to the placebo (3).).

Review of Chapter 2

- Antioxidants protect the body from free radicals, decrease chronic inflammation, and may reduce the risk of a multitude of chronic diseases and conditions.
- Antioxidants appear to positively impact mood and may reduce the risk and/or severity of depression, anxiety, and stress.
- Antioxidant-rich foods including fruits, vegetables, nuts, seeds, whole grains, tea, dark chocolate, rosemary, sage, and garlic have been associated with a reduced risk of depression, anxiety, and stress.
- Omega-3 may play a role in reducing the risk and symptoms of mood disorders like depression and anxiety and may help with feelings of stress. Omega-3 can be found in freshwater fish, nuts, and seeds.
- Research shows that diets high in whole foods, vegetables, fruit, fish, whole grains, lean meats, nuts, seeds, legumes, salmon, tuna, green tea, herbs, and spices and low in ultra-processed foods, sugary foods, trans fat, and energy-dense, low nutrient foods are more likely to provide protection against mental disorders. In other words, the higher the quality of the diet, the less likely you will experience depression (47, 112).
- To eat a diet that promotes cognitive function, eat mostly plant-based whole foods and consist of antioxidant and Omega-3-rich foods. Include vegetables, especially leafy

greens, nuts, seeds, fruits, berries, beans, whole grains, fish, poultry, olive oil, green team, and dark chocolate.

- Limit foods that promote cognitive decline when eaten in excess, like refined carbohydrates and sugars, ultra-processed foods, processed meats, and fried foods.
- Incorporate probiotics and prebiotics into your diet.
- Add Turmeric, Rosemary, and Sage to some of your meals.

Chapter 3: The "Right" Foods and Essential Nutrients for the Body

When we are talking about nutrition for the body, we are talking about foods that protect our bodies from chronic disease, help improve longevity, and help us feel energetic. These foods will also help with mobility. For example, when I changed my diet, I saw a significant improvement in my mobility. I could do things in my 40s that I couldn't do in my late 20s. I found that I had more energy and mobility to play on the playground with my children, and I could quickly and easily pick up my children's toys from the floor. I could dance with my daughter and run with my soccer-playing son, albeit I was much slower than he.

Now let's touch on what the research says about how food can promote a healthy body.

Food and Cancer Prevention

Antioxidants and Cancer Prevention

According to research, 30-35% of cancer cases are linked to diet. Excess weight is also linked to a 50% increased risk of developing cancer (94). Plant-based diets high in vegetables, whole grains, nuts, seeds, legumes, olive oil, and green tea; moderate in fish, like salmon; and moderate-to-low in lean meats have been shown to reduce cancer cell growth and the risk developing of cancer (78).

Fruits and vegetable consumption appears crucial in regard to reducing the risk of cancer. Diets high in fruits and vegetables decrease the risk of breast cancer, colorectal cancer, prostate cancer around 60-70%, and lung cancer by 40-50%, according to one review (78). In a small human trial, people with colon cancer saw a 7% reduction in cancer growth after consuming bilberry extract for seven days. In an animal study, raspberries reduced esophageal tumor incidence by 54% and decreased the number of tumors by 62% (61).

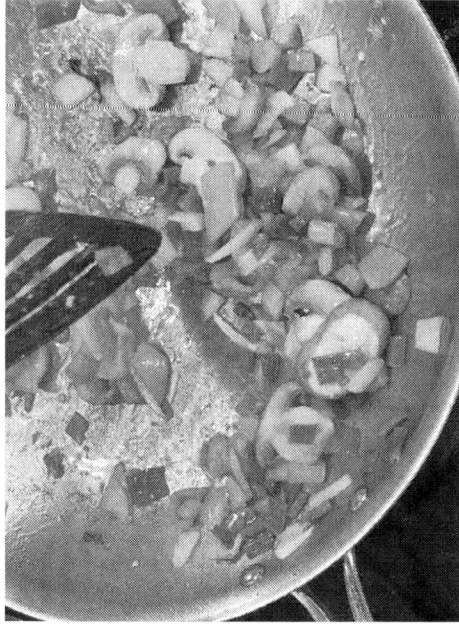

Sulforaphane is found in vegetables like broccoli and broccoli sprouts. Sulforaphane may reduce the size and number of some cancers cells by 50-75%, according to some in vitro research (69, 117).

Fruits and vegetables are not the only antioxidant-rich foods; they may help prevent cancer. Nuts and seeds show promise as well. High nuts consumption is associated with decreased prevalence of cancer and death from cancer, based on results from a systemic review (131). In another study, mice given walnuts saw an 80% decrease in the growth rate of breast cancer and a 60% reduction in the number of cancer cells (38).

Based on research, spices containing antioxidants may have anti-cancer properties as well. Spices showing promise include garlic, turmeric, cinnamon, and rosemary (5, 6, 19, 90, 97).

The bottom line is there is strong research showing that foods high in antioxidants significantly reduce the risk of cancer and, along with treatment, may even help in the cancer fight once someone has developed cancer. Anti-cancer antioxidant-rich foods include:

- Vegetables, especially broccoli, broccoli sprouts, and dark leafy greens.
- Fruit, especially berries, nuts.
- Seeds.
- Spices, especially turmeric, garlic, rosemary, and cinnamon.

Probiotics and Cancer Prevention

Probiotics may help with cancer prevention, according to both animal and human studies. Probiotics may even have an anti-cancer effect in patients who already have cancer (94).

High intakes of refined carbohydrates and sugar, as well as ultra-processed foods, fried foods, processed meats, and smoked meats, may increase the risk of cancer. These foods are also associated with poor gut health.

Food and Neurodegenerative Diseases

Neurodegenerative diseases are diseases in which degeneration of the nervous symptoms occurs. Much of this degeneration occurs in the neurons in the brain but can affect the whole body. For example, Alzheimer's is considered a neurodegenerative disease.

Other neurodegenerative diseases include ALS and Parkinson's disease. ALS affects the motor neurons of the spinal cord and causes progressive weakness and atrophy of muscles. Although more research is needed, several studies, including a systemic review, point to poor gut health as one contributing factor of ALS (14, 77, 130).

Antioxidants may be helpful in the prevention of ALS as well. According to 5 studies, diets high in antioxidant-rich foods are associated with a reduced risk of developing ALS (29). Remember, prebiotics and probiotics are helpful when it comes to promoting gut health.

Parkinson's is another neurodegenerative disease in which the basal ganglia of the brain begin to degenerate. People with Parkinson's also have a deficiency of dopamine. Tremors and muscle rigidity throughout the body are characteristics of Parkinson's disease. Although more human studies are needed, in vitro studies show probiotics decrease inflammation and bacterial overgrowth found in individuals with Parkinson's disease (120).

Food and Autoimmune Diseases

Tip 25: Eat foods that contain antioxidants, omega-3, probiotics, prebiotics, and vitamin D.

These substances may reduce the risk of developing autoimmune diseases.

Autoimmune diseases are diseases that can affect the immune system of our body. Although autoimmune diseases appear to be genetic, certain triggers in our diet and lifestyle may contribute to the development of autoimmune diseases.

Below is a List of Common Autoimmune Diseases:

- Type 1 Diabetes
- Vasculitis
- Rheumatoid arthritis
- Multiple Sclerosis (MS)
- Hashimoto's Disease
- Psoriasis
- Irritable Bowel Disease (IBD)
- Henoch-Schoenlein purpura (HSP)
- Crohn's Disease
- Lupus

Antioxidants and Autoimmune Diseases

In general, antioxidant-rich diets like the Mediterranean diet have been linked to an expanded lifespan and reduced symptoms of some autoimmune diseases like Rheumatoid Arthritis. The Mediterranean diet is known for being a diet high in fruits and vegetables, including leafy greens, nuts, seeds, and fish, and low in sugar, high fructose corn syrup, processed food, trans fat, vegetable oils, refined carbohydrates, processed meats, and excessive alcohol (103).

Tip 26: Limit your sugar intake by choosing sauces and condiments labeled "no sugar added." You can find "No Sugar added" ketchup, BBQ sauce, tomato sauce, and salad dressings, to name a few.

Higher vegetables and consequently higher antioxidant consumption reduced the rate of MS. In fact, a one-cup increase in vegetable intakes, excluding the nightshade vegetables, decreased the rate of relapse of MS by 50%. Potatoes and legumes are examples of nightshade vegetables (56).

Inversely, diets low in antioxidants and high in inflammatory foods may promote autoimmune diseases. Ultra-processed foods, processed meats with nitrates and nitrites, trans fat, refined carbohydrates, and sugar are pro-inflammatory foods, so consider only eating these foods occasionally (73).

Tip 27: When you do eat processed meats, like luncheon meats, look for lean turkey, labeled "No nitrate/nitrite added" and "No Sugar added."

Luncheon meats are considered processed meats. No nitrate/nitrite added lean turkey slices are one of the best options.

Probiotics and Autoimmune Diseases

Remember, autoimmune diseases occur when the immune system is not working properly. For forty years, animal and human studies have shown a link between probiotic intakes and positive effects on immunity and autoimmune diseases (56, 71).

According to several studies, including the gold standard, randomized-controlled studies, probiotics may improve GI symptoms and inflammation in Rheumatoid Arthritis, Ulcerative Colitis, and Multiple Sclerosis and help with symptoms in individuals with Lupus. In addition, a meta-analysis showed probiotics might have a positive impact on Irritable Bowel Diseases, including Crohn's disease and ulcerative colitis. Probiotics may even slow the progression of IBS, ulcerative colitis, and Crohn's disease (51, 56, 71, 98). Remember, prebiotic fiber is also important for gut health and should be included in your diet.

Multiple Sclerosis (MS) and Diet

We have established that antioxidants and probiotics may help reduce the risk of developing Multiple Sclerosis, but there are a few other nutrients that may be beneficial.

Other factors that may increase the risk of developing Multiple Sclerosis are vitamin D deficiency, low sun exposure (which can cause vitamin D deficiency), viral exposure, and obesity. For example, researchers have observed that if you were born below 35-degree latitude and lived there for the first ten years of your life, your risk of developing Multiple Sclerosis is reduced by 50%. This may be due to people in these areas getting more vitamin d from sun exposure (89). Another study showed that when individuals took vitamin D supplements, their risk of developing Multiple Sclerosis decreased by 40% (89).

According to a review, calorie restriction, healthy fats, and green tea extract (an antioxidant) may help reduce symptoms of Multiple Sclerosis, whereas diets high in saturated fat and salt may worsen Multiple Sclerosis symptoms.

Rheumatoid Arthritis and Diet

Extensive evidence, including randomized controlled studies (the gold standard of studies), indicates that Omega-3 supplements significantly slow the progression of Rheumatoid Arthritis (103).

A Note on Gluten and Autoimmune Diseases

People with Celiac disease must always avoid gluten; however, a gluten-free or at least a temporarily gluten-free diet may also be beneficial to those suffering from another autoimmune disease if they are sensitive to gluten (63).

Talk with your doctor or a dietitian if you think you may be sensitive to gluten or any other food, as foods in which you are intolerant or sensitive may exasperate your autoimmune disease.

Food, Asthma, and Seasonal Allergies

Tip 28: To relieve symptoms of seasonal allergies and asthma, include omega-3, antioxidants, vitamin D, and probiotics in your daily diet.

The big four when it comes to foods that can help asthma and seasonal allergies are omega-3, antioxidants, vitamin D, and probiotics.

Omega-3, Asthma, and Seasonal Allergies

Most research supports the theory that omega-3 is helpful in the prevention and treatment of seasonal allergies. In addition, high omega-3 consumption is associated with better asthma control (82, 121).

Antioxidants, Asthma, and Seasonal Allergies

While an array of antioxidants protects from seasonal allergy and asthma symptoms, the antioxidant quercetin appears particularly important for allergy and asthma management.

One study looked at 13,000 adults and found that apples and pears are positively associated with lung function. Apples, which are a good source of quercetin, have a stronger inverse link to asthma than total fruit and vegetable consumption (16)!

Vitamin D, Asthma, and Seasonal Allergies

According to some research, Vitamin D supplementation may reduce the severity of asthma attacks by about 31-36% in people with asthma and may even reduce the number of asthma emergency room visits, according to some research (34).

Probiotics, Asthma, and Seasonal Allergies

According to research, probiotics may help prevent seasonal allergies and protect us from asthma triggers by improving the protectiveness of the gut. Are you noticing a pattern? Probiotics keep showing up on the list, and here they are again. Probiotics may help ward off seasonal allergies and reduce the frequency of asthma attacks, according to several studies and systemic reviews (55).

Food and Immunity: Can Food Keep You from Getting Sick as Often?

Tip 29: During the cold and flu season, consider increasing your intake of zinc, vitamin D, and vitamin C. Talk with your doctor before taking any supplements.

While food can't boost the immune system, it can support the immune system so that your immune system can function at optimal levels

Getting sick often can put your whole life on a standstill for days, if not weeks, but when your immune system is functioning optimally, you may notice you are not getting sick as often.

Several nutrients and substances promote healthy immune function. One of those is antioxidants. Extensive research indicated that the antioxidants ECGC, anthocyanin, Selenium, Quercetin, Vitamin A, Vitamin E, Vitamin C, and zinc had been shown to have antiviral and antibacterial properties. Antioxidants may even reduce the frequency of upper respiratory symptoms. Polyphenols have also been shown to reduce the severity of cold and flu symptoms (28, 91, 95, 107, 114, 115). According to a review, flavonoid supplements reduced upper respiratory infections by 33% and decreased the number of sick days by 40% (118). ECGC catechins are an antioxidant in green tea, and these ECGC catechins may reduce the symptoms of the common cold by 31.1% and the duration of a cold by 30.6% based on research (30).

Vitamin C may be the most well-known immune-supportive antioxidant vitamin for a good reason. Although regularly taking vitamin C supplements does not appear to prevent the common cold in the general population, it does appear to shorten the duration (109). Vitamin C may, however, prevent the common cold in those who participate in strenuous physical activity like marathon runners. Therefore, these athletes need more vitamin C than the general population.

Zinc is a mineral that acts as an antioxidant and is needed for optimal immune function. Adequate zinc helps increase white blood cell count and helps fight infection. Thus, zinc is a crucial mineral in regard to the immune system (109, 116). According to various research articles, taking zinc supplements may shorten the duration of a cold by 33-44% (109).

Foods that are high in antioxidants, as well as antioxidant-rich spices, are perfect editions to your healthy diet. In addition, spices like turmeric, garlic, ginger, rosemary, and cinnamon have been shown to have antiviral properties (20, 87, 128).

A systemic review suggests that garlic lowered the risk of getting the common cold by 63% and shortened the duration of a cold by 70%

compared to the placebo. Furthermore, for those who did get the cold, the duration was 70% shorter when compared to the placebo groups (70).

Vitamin D is another vital immune-supportive vitamin. People with vitamin D deficiency are more at risk of catching a cold, flu, and respiratory infections (18, 84, 109).

Probiotics and the Immune System

Since 70% of the immune system lives in the GI tract; then it may come as no surprise to hear probiotics may help reduce the frequency and severity of communal diseases (17, 54, 67, 92, 125, 126). Although studies on both humans and animals show that probiotics positively impact immunity, one of the most fascinating studies is a mice study (54, 66, 92, 126). In this study, mice were fed a lethal dose of parainfluenza. Then, some of the mice were given a probiotic while others were not. The mice taking the probiotic had a 61% survival rate. The mice who did not take probiotics had a 0% survival rate.

A review of 12 studies also found that people who took probiotics had less frequent and shorter upper respiratory infections.

Can Certain Foods Help Me Live Longer?

Tip 30: Eat mostly plant-based meals.

When you are looking for research on what to eat to promote long life, look no further than the Blue Zone research. The Blue Zones refers to areas in the world where people are living longer, higher-quality lives than many of us in the rest of the world.

The Blue Zones Include:

- Okinawa, Japan
- Loma Linda, CA
- Nicoya, Costa Rica
- Sardinia, Italy
- Ikaria, Greece

The diets of the people living in these Blue Zones are similar even though they all come from different areas of the world and different cultural backgrounds. These similarities in their diets are now referred to by many as the Blue Zone Diet. The Blue Zone diet is mostly plant-based (around 90-100% plant-based). The diet consists of mostly fruits, vegetables, fish, legumes, nuts, seeds, whole grains, and olive oil. When they do eat animal protein, the common choice is often fish.

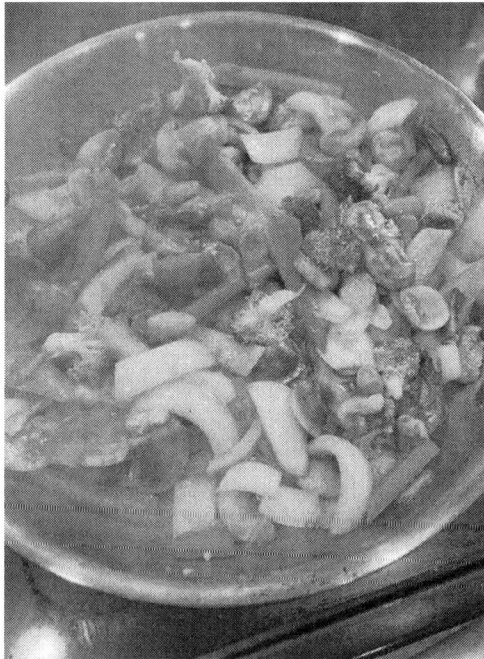

Review of Chapter 3

- The "right" foods for the body essentially mean foods that promote longevity, improve mobility and energy levels, and reduce the risk of chronic diseases and conditions.
- Plant-based diets high in antioxidant-rich fruits and vegetables, as well as probiotics and prebiotics, reduce the risk of some cancers, neurodegenerative diseases, autoimmune diseases, asthma, and seasonal allergies.
- These anti-inflammatory foods will also promote mobility and energy.
- Omega-3 and vitamin D are also anti-inflammatory and may reduce the risk of developing some autoimmune diseases.
- Immune supportive nutrients include vitamin C, vitamin D, zinc, antioxidants, and probiotics.
- People living in the Blue Zones tend to live longer lives and are less likely to develop chronic diseases and conditions. Their diets are 90-100% plant-based and consist of mostly fruits, vegetables, nuts, seeds, legumes, whole grains, and olive oil.

Chapter 4: Will Weight Loss Help Me Become a Healthier Person?

Does weight actually impact our health? Recent studies have questioned whether weight really plays as big of a part in our health as we once thought. For example, some studies had demonstrated that when individuals began to eat healthier, their labs and medical conditions improved regardless of whether they lost weight or not (76, 127).

Studies like these have dietitians, doctors, and scientists wondering whether healthy behaviors, not weight, determine someone's health. Yet, other studies show that weight and excessive calorie intake impact some conditions such as mobility, joint pain, shortness of breath, and motor and cognitive function. For example, reducing calories by 40% improved motor and cognitive function associated with aging (74).

So, Does Weight Actually Impact Our Health?

Weight does not appear to be the only or even the major factor in health like we once thought, but weight can affect our health. However, you don't have to look like a supermodel to be extremely healthy. In fact, the supermodel physique will be healthy for some and not for others.

For me, I lost weight when I stopped focusing on weight and started focusing on health, and I encourage my clients to try this approach as well. You will often find when you eat healthier; your body will naturally fall into the size that is optimal for you.

Furthermore, weight loss goals depend on what you are trying to achieve. For example, weight goals will be different for someone who wants to simply reduce the risk of chronic disease than it would be for someone who wants to improve their speed and athleticism for a sport.

But if weight changes are part of your "becoming a healthier person" goals, then what are the best strategies you can incorporate to achieve your weight goals?

How Does Eating Healthier Naturally Help with Weight Loss Goals When Weight Loss May Be Beneficial?

Tip 31: For weight loss goals, eat protein-rich food (it can be plant-based) at every meal.

Protein takes more energy to digest and promotes feelings of satiety.

Weight loss usually occurs when we are eating fewer calories than we are using. Eating filling foods helps us eat less because...well...we are full. A healthy diet focuses on eating more vegetables. Vegetables are lower in calories and higher in super-filling fiber. Speaking of fiber, fiber foods, as well as protein foods, spicy foods, hot foods, and soup, help your body feel full.

Tip 32: Eat fiber at every meal to help you feel full and satisfied.

Whole grains vs. refined grains are going to promote weight loss because of the high fiber content in whole grains. On the other hand, refined carbohydrates and sugar are low in fiber and cause your blood sugar levels to spike, then crash, leaving you hungry for more food.

Other Tips for Weight Loss:

Tip 33: Eat more whole foods and less processed foods.

The body must work harder and use more energy (i.e., calories) to process whole foods.

Tip 34: Drink plenty of water.

Being only 1-2% dehydrated can slow metabolism,

Tip 35: Add capsaicin-rich foods like peppers to some of your meals.

Studies show capsaicin may slightly increase metabolism (50).

Tip 36: Add flavor to a salad with lighter options like lemon juice, vinegar, and olive oil.

Tip 37: Instead of frying, cook foods by baking, steaming, microwaving, or stir-frying in a light coating of healthy oil like avocado oil.

Tip 38: If you are going to a potluck party, bring your own nourishing dish to eat and share with others.

If you bring a healthy dish, you know you will have a healthy option no matter what everyone else brings.

Tip 39: Don't overdo the alcohol.

Alcohol leaves you feeling sluggish ad weak the next day, plus alcohol lowers your inhibitions. You might find it easier to binge eat after a few too many mixed drinks. Not to mention, most alcoholic drinks provide empty calories.

Tip 40: Bring your food to work on most days.

Restaurants usually promote overeating and often have less nutritious options. Eating out often can also cause a financial strain because dining out can get expensive. When you bring your food from home, you have more control over what you put into your body.

Mindful Eating for Weight Maintenance, Weight Loss, and Weight Gain Needs

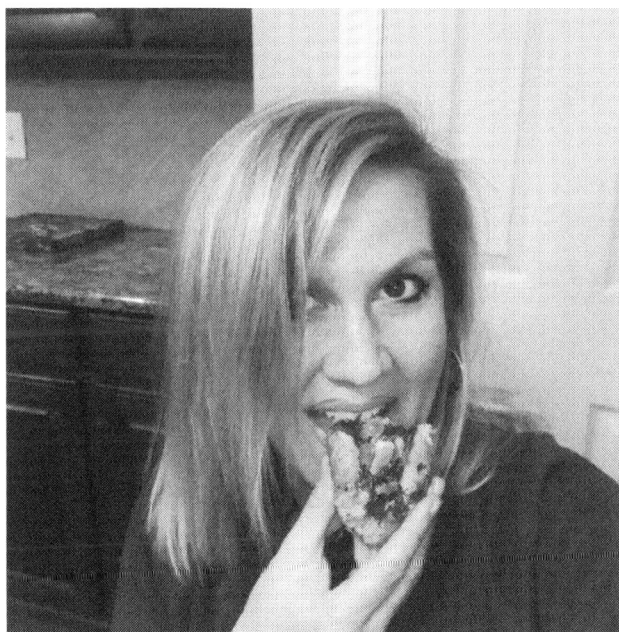

Regardless of whether you hope to lose weight, gain weight, or maintain weight, portion awareness through mindful eating is one of the best techniques for weight management.

Imagine for a moment that you are about to eat your food, but before you start, you take a moment to notice everything about the meal in front of you. You notice the smell, the colors, and the shapes of the food on your plate.

Tip 41: Make your plate look pretty.

The more attractive your plate is, the more satisfied with your meal you will feel. Our eating experience starts when we look at and smell our food. To make your plate look appealing, leave "white space." In other words, don't pile your food onto the plate. Instead, leave space between your food and around the outer rim. This helps with portions as well.

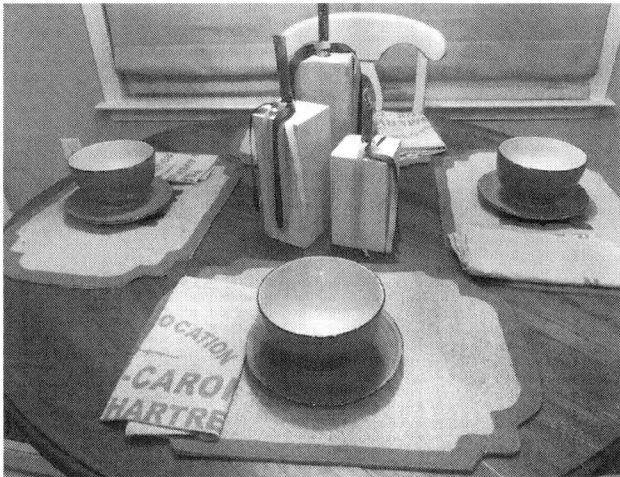

Now that you have plated your food, it is time to pause and think about the food you are about to eat. Look at your food and think about the nutrients that particular food contains. Then, take a moment to appreciate what that food does for your body. When you think about the benefits of nourishing foods, you will notice that you begin to desire nourishing foods. Your mindset and cravings begin to shift.

After you have visually taken in the food in front of you, you are ready to taste your first bite. While that bite is in your mouth, focus on the flavors and textures in that bite. While you are chewing, you put your fork down. You don't begin preparing your next bite until you have completely finished the bite in your mouth. Once you are done with that first bite, you cleanse your palette with water and start the eating process all over again.

This is what mindful eating looks like. It may seem strange, but I encourage you to give it a try. You will be surprised at how incredibly full you will begin to feel as you mindfully eat. Mindful eating helps you notice your hunger cues and feel physically and emotionally satisfied when your body is ready to stop eating.

Tip 42: Put your fork down in between bites.

Pick it up only after you have completely swallowed the food in your mouth.

Tip 43: Take a sip of water between every bite to cleanse your palette and slow down the eating process.

Mindful eating also involves listening to your hunger cues. What signal is your body trying to communicate with you when you are hungry? Signals of hunger include growling or empty feelings in your stomach, low energy, and food cravings. When you have gone too long without eating, you may experience a headache or even feelings of nausea.

When you are full, your energy feels restored. Your stomach is no longer growling, and other hunger symptoms have gone away. This is usually where your body feels at its best. Finally, your body has the food it needs to seize the day.

When you are overly full, your stomach feels distended. You may have moved past feeling energetic and now feel heavy and tired. When you eat more slowly and pause throughout the meal, you give yourself time to notice these signals.

In my experience, this has been one of the best ways to naturally eat the number of calories your body is supposed to eat. You do not need willpower or cheat days because you are always emotionally and physically enjoying your food.

Other Tips That May Help with Mindful Eating

Tip 44: Sit down when you eat.

Standing up promotes mindless eating. Instead, sit down and enjoy your food. When you sit down, you can more fully notice your body's hunger/full signals.

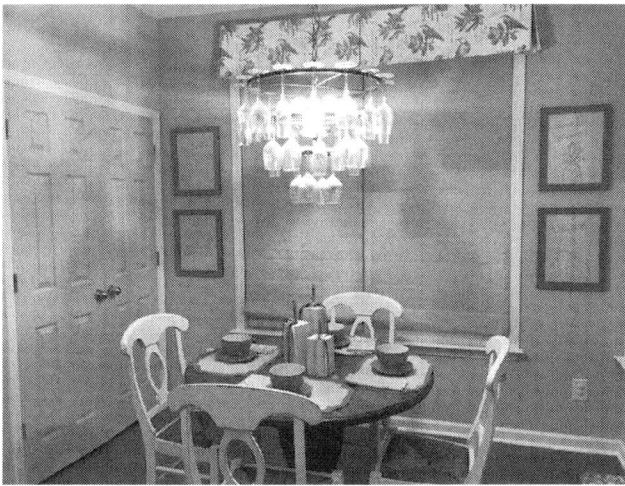

Tip 45: Stop doing other things like surfing the internet or watching TV while eating.

Doing other things discourages mindful eating. For example, you may want to try turning off the TV so that you can pay attention to the flavors in your food.

Other Tips That May Help with Portions

Tip 46: Eat from a smaller breakfast plate instead of a dinner plate.

Dinner plates are usually larger than many need.

Tip 47: Restaurants usually give us much more than we actually need.

Ask the waiter to bring a to-go box when he brings your meal. Before you begin eating, fill your to-go box until your plate no longer looks over-the-top.

Tip 48: Limit the number of sides you cook.

We tend to overeat when we have too many options. For example, if you made a meatloaf, rice and gravy, fried okra, buttered biscuit, and a fruit cobbler for dinner, even if you put a small amount of each of these on your plate, your plate would still be piled high with food. There is no way to include all of these sides onto a small dinner plate with ample "white space."

Tip 49: Drink water before a meal and with meals.

To feel satisfied, we must feed our thirst along with our hunger.

Tip 50: Freeze or refrigerate your food after you have finished cooking and plating your food.

This may help with the desire to mindlessly nibble on seconds after you are full. Plus, clean-up is already done! So you can enjoy your meal without worrying about cleaning up

Tip 51: Wait 10 or 15 minutes before going back for seconds.

Sometimes it takes our body a moment to notice whether we are full or not. Waiting before going for seconds gives your body a chance to notice your hunger cues. You might not want seconds after all.

Tip 52: Keep the serving dishes off the dinner table.

When it is time to eat, serve your food from the kitchen, not the dinner table. It is just a little easier to mindlessly grab more food even when you are full if the food is sitting in front of you at the dinner table.

Tip 53: When at a party, decide on your top 5 favorite dishes and eat those.

Parties often provide more food choices than we could ever fit onto our plate. If we overeat, then we are left feeling sluggish for the rest of the party. If there are just too many choices, try choosing your top five. Then, mindfully enjoy your absolute favorites.

Tip 54: At restaurants, choose baked or grilled dishes instead of fried, and choose lean turkey, chicken, fish, or vegetarian options.

These options tend to be higher in filling nutrients and lower in empty calories.

Tip 56: When eating out, choose a vegetable option instead of less nutritious sides like French fries.

This one small change can have a huge impact on the calories and nutrients in your meal.

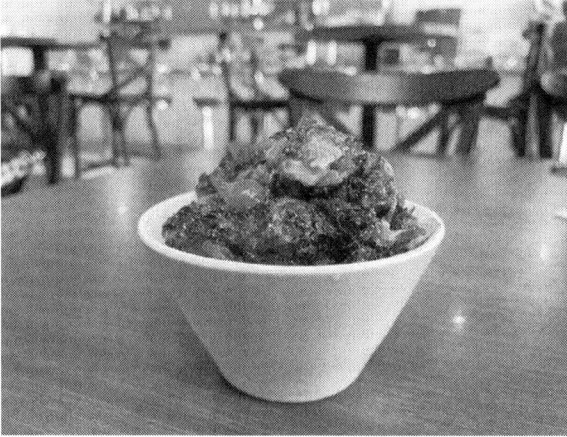

Tip 57: If you know you are just too busy to cook, then look for healthy pre-packaged meal options.

Look for packages that contain vegetables, whole grains, and lean meats. Check the back label. Look for packaged food with less added sugar, zero trans-fat, and whole-food ingredients.

Tip 58: Ask for water at restaurants.

Refills of sugary drinks can have a huge impact on your calorie and sugar intake. For example, just three refills of a sugary soda are around 500 calories alone!

Emotional Eating

Sometimes we eat because food soothes our emotions. For example, we may crave food when we are bored, stressed, tired, procrastinating, or sad. I am going to tell you something you may not have heard before. Sometimes emotional eating is okay. That food soothes your soul. Food should bring us nourishment and joy. The problem with emotional eating is that we sometimes binge eat or overeat. I recommend trying other ways to self-soothe first, but if it doesn't work, then mindfully eat.

Tip 59: Make a list of activities you enjoy doing when you are feeling bored, stressed, sad, or need a break.

When you feel like trying to emotionally eat, do something from your list instead. Self-soothing ideas:

- Read a book.
- Take a hot bath.
- Take a short nap.
- Write in your journal.
- Sit on your porch with a calming green tea or kombucha.
- Go for a walk.
- Watch something on TV.

Tip 60: When you emotionally eat, make sure you are still practicing mindful eating.

Mindful eating is also relaxing and stress relieving because you are taking the time to slow down. Mindful eating also helps prevent binges.

Tip 61: Make sure you regularly include the foods that help reduce the risk or symptoms of depression, stress, and anxiety in your diet.

Go back to chapter 2 to review which foods that help mood.

Tip 62: Talk with your doctor about adding a supplement listed in the Mood section of chapter 7 to your routine.

Note: If you are experiencing severe depression, anxiety, or have other concerns about your mood, talk with your doctor right away. Sometimes medical treatment is needed.

What We Have Learned So Far

Before we go any further, let's remind ourselves what we are trying to learn from this book. After reading this book, we want to understand what the "right" foods to eat are in order to take in all the essential nutrients and become a healthier person. The answer to this question is that the "right foods" to eat are the foods that will positively impact the whole person- the mind and body. These are foods that will reduce the risk of chronic diseases and conditions, promote optimal brain function, support the immune system, and help our mood. These foods will also help lead us to the weight that is best for our bodies.

The "perfect" diet will vary among individuals, which is why getting private counseling from a dietitian is helpful. However, based on this research, some of the best foods to eat to get in all of the powerful essential nutrients and become a healthier person are vegetables, fruit, nuts, seeds, whole grains, fish, tea, dark chocolate, and fresh herbs and spices. So now we know what to eat, but how do we get all of these foods into our diets?

Review of Chapter 4

- While weight is one factor that contributes to our overall health, it may not be the major contributing factor when it comes to our health. Therefore, we should focus more on eating for nourishment more than on weight desires.
- Mindful eating helps stabilize weight by promoting feelings of fullness and satisfaction after eating. Mindful eating helps when we are eating at home, a restaurant, or at a party and even helps when applied to emotional eating.
- Eating high protein and fiber foods helps us feel full as well.
- Fiber-rich foods include whole grains, fruits, vegetables, nuts, and seeds.

- Eating plenty of vegetables at every meal and for snacks helps with weight loss because vegetables are both low in calories and high in fiber.

Chapter 5: What Can I Do to Become a Healthier Person?

The amount of food a person should eat will vary based on height, weight, and lifestyle. You can find out your personal needs from a local dietitian, or you can focus on listening to your body through mindful eating. (Remember, your body gives signals, and if you listen to those signals, you will often naturally eat the amount your body needs). However, you can use the following guidelines to make sure you are eating the essential nutrients needed to become a healthier person:

Tip 63: Revamp your kitchen. Remove or donate the less nutrient-dense foods and stock your kitchen with foods that meet the guidelines below.

Meal Guidelines for Healthy Eating

- Eat mostly plant-based meals.

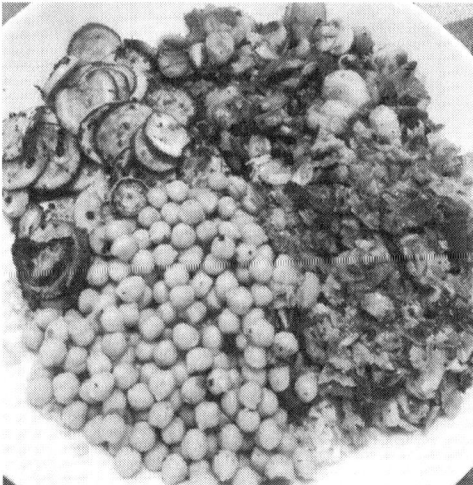

Tip 64: You can incorporate a more plant-based lifestyle by either making more of your meals meat-free or making the meat portions smaller on your plate.

Of course, you can also decide to fully embrace the vegetarian or pescatarian lifestyle. Pescatarian means you are a vegetarian, except you also eat fish.

- Eat whole grains two to three times a day (If you are gluten intolerant or have Celiac disease, make sure you eat gluten-free whole grains)

Whole grains include brown rice, quinoa, whole-wheat pasta, whole-wheat pizza crust, Whole-wheat tortillas, oats, buckwheat, and popcorn.

Carbohydrates are often used as the base for our meals. A base is a food we use to hold the other food. For instance, pasta is the base for spaghetti because you put the sauce, vegetables, or meat on top of the pasta. Another example would be a sandwich. The bread (a carbohydrate) is the "thing" that holds the other ingredients. Other carbohydrate bases would be pizza crust, pie crust, rice, tortillas, and wraps.

Although we don't have to go low carb, we can do some things to prevent excessive carb intake. Carbs may traditionally be the base of a meal, but they don't have to be.

Below are a few alternative base tips:

Tip 65: Sometimes, use cauliflower rice instead of rice.

This doesn't mean never eating brown rice. Brown rice is a healthy whole grain, but you can add variety and increase your vegetable intake by using cauliflower rice for some of your meals.

Tip 66: Sometimes, use zoodles, konjac noodles, or palmini instead of pasta.

Unless you have Celiac disease or are gluten intolerant/sensitive, whole-wheat pasta is a healthy option; however, in the name of variety, you can also use alternative pasta like zoodles, konjac noodles, or palmini noodles.

Tip 67: On occasion, make lettuce wraps instead of traditional wraps.

Lettuce wraps are another fun way to change up the traditional wraps. Remember, when you do eat grain wraps, choose the whole grain varieties.

Tip 68: Eat soup sometimes.

Can you guess what the base would be in a soup? Did you guess the liquid? The liquid is considered the base because it holds all the other ingredients.

Tip 69: Eat more salads with leafy greens.

In this option, the leafy greens are the base for your meal.

Tip 70: Make pizza using cloud bread on occasion (See recipe in chapter 8).

You can always make pizza using a whole grain crust, but whole-grain pie crust is sometimes hard to find. This cloud bread recipe is an excellent pizza crust option.

Tip 71: To cut down on excessive carbs, make vegetables the star of your meal instead of carbohydrates.

You don't have to eat low carb to eat healthily, but we may have been eating excessive carbs in the past. For example, eating a plate filled with pasta and two large pieces of garlic bread was not uncommon a few years ago and even today. This type of eating provides more carbohydrates than most people need. At restaurants, many people find themselves eating all of the breadbaskets before the meal arrives. This is another example of what may be considered excessive carbs for most people.

Tip 72: You can also cut down on excessive carbs by eating a sandwich open-faced.

An open-faced sandwich is when you put the toppings on one slice of bread, but you leave off the top piece of bread. This will cut down on calories as well.

Tip 73: When you go out to eat, you may want to ask the server to hold the breadbasket.

I don't know about you, but when I am hungry and waiting for food, I can eat two baskets of bread all by my lonesome. But if I want to enjoy my meal instead of getting full before it arrives, then I simply ask my server not to bring the basket.

- Eat vegetables at every meal.

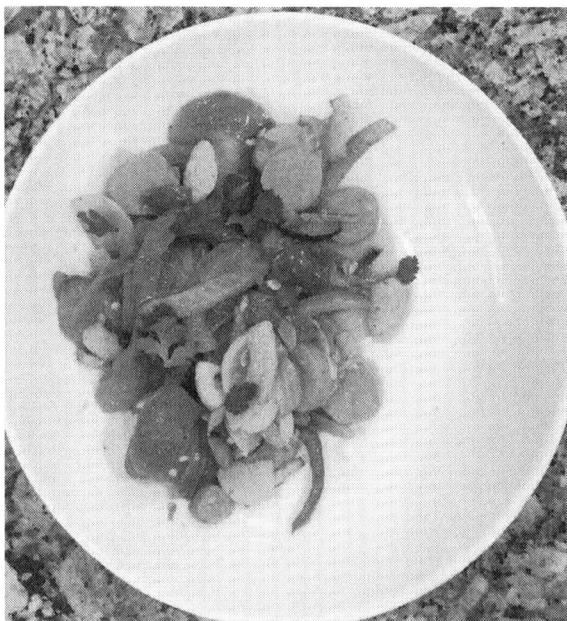

Tip 74: Make sure dark leafy greens are included once a day.

Remember from chapters 2 and 3 that dark leafy greens are powerhouse vegetables and full of incredible antioxidants.

Tip 75: Add vegetables to your existing recipes.

When you add vegetables to your recipes, you will have more nutrients and fewer calories per serving. For example, one cup of spaghetti without vegetables will have more calories than 1 cup of spaghetti filled with mushrooms, onions, carrots, and spinach.

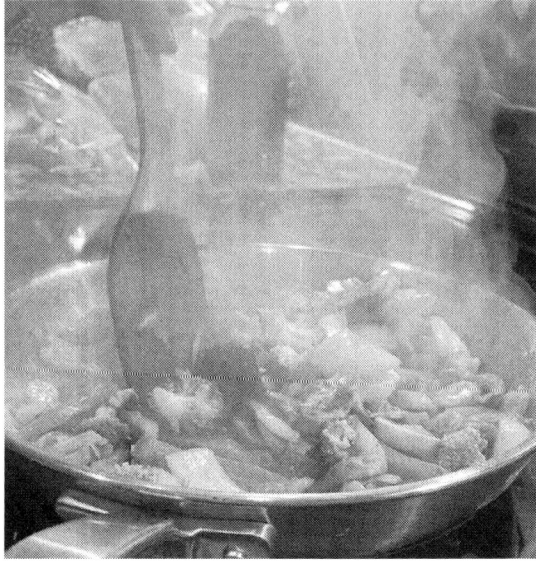

- Eat nuts and seeds around five times per week.

Tip 76: Add nuts and berries to your yogurt for breakfast, or eat a handful of nuts as a snack.

Adding nuts to your diet can sometimes be tricky. They are not often seen in many lunch and dinner recipes. You can, however, add nuts to your yogurt at breakfast or just eat a handful for a snack. Plus, the yogurt provides probiotics and protein as well.

Tip 77: You can also add a variety of nuts and seeds to a Pesto Recipe (See Chapter 8 for the recipe.)

The pesto recipe in this book is a nutrient powerhouse. This recipe contains antioxidants, fiber, protein, and ALA Omega-3 all in one creamy, delicious sauce.

Tip 78: Nuts and seeds can easily be sprinkled over a salad to add a crunch while simultaneously adding healthy fats, fiber, protein, and antioxidants.

This is such a simple trick for sneaking nuts and seeds into your regular meals.

- Eat beans and legumes around four times a week.

Tip 79: Throw beans into a soup or mix them with whole-grain to add protein to a plant-based meal.

Mostly-plant based doesn't mean low in protein. Beans (as well as nuts and seeds) are a perfect protein alternative to animal protein.

- Eat poultry, like turkey or chicken, two times a week (unless you are a vegetarian or pescatarian)

Tip 80: Get creative with your meals. Use chicken breast, turkey slices, ground chicken, ground turkey, or canned chicken to add lean meats to your meals.

Tuna, salmon, and chicken pouches or cans are such a quick and easy way to add protein as well. They don't even require cooking.

- Eat fish two times a week.

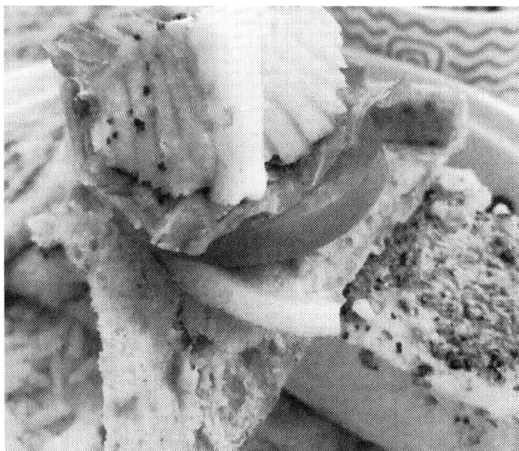

Tip 81: Include Omega-3-rich fish like salmon or tuna.

I like to look for salmon options when I am dining out. I also like to keep frozen salmon in my fridge. Frozen salmon is easy to bake, sauté, or air fry. I also keep pouches or cans of salmon and tuna in my pantry. I just throw them on my salad when I want to add a little protein and omega-3 to my dark leafy greens.

Tip 82: Look for wild-caught, low mercury fish. You can find frozen, canned, or pouches of tuna or salmon labeled wild-caught and low mercury.

- Eat fruit once a day and make sure that fruit is a berry at least two times a week.

Tip 84: Eat berries in a smoothie, as part of a trail mix, in a yogurt parfait, or on top of a fresh summer salad.

Like nuts, sometimes you must get creative when it comes to adding berries to your recipes. Berries are fantastic in salads, smoothies, and trail mixes.

- Eat probiotic and prebiotic-rich foods 4 to 5 times a week.

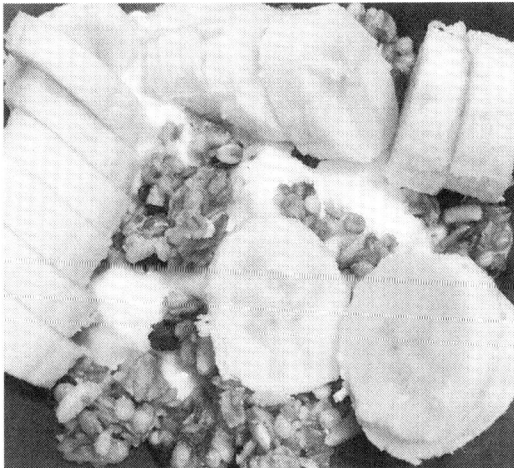

Tip 85: Make those berry smoothies or parfaits using probiotic-rich yogurt.

Add nuts and seeds like chia, hemp, or flaxseeds, and you have packed your parfait with antioxidants, fiber, probiotics, ALA Omega-3s, vitamins, minerals, and protein.

Meal Planning Tips

Now you know the guidelines; the next step is figuring out how to make your daily meals follow these guidelines.

Tip 86: One way to make sure your daily meals meet the above guidelines is to search for Mediterranean diet recipes, Blue Zone recipes, Prudent diet recipes, Pescatarian recipes, and MIND diet recipes on the web.

The diets follow the healthy guidelines listed in this book.

Tip 87: You can also search for Mediterranean, Blue Zone, Pescatarian, and MIND cookbooks and make your meals using the recipes from the cookbooks.

Cookbooks are also a great option because they provide a group of recipes in one nicely organized location.

Note: You can find a meal plan and fantastic recipes that meet the guidelines listed above at the back of this book.

Tip 88: If you are trying to make a meal on your own, simply think of your favorite meals but change them by adding in more vegetables or substituting your normal meat with lean meat. You can also substitute any of your grains with the whole grain version.

Take classic spaghetti, for example. Instead of using regular pasta, you could use whole grain or add more vegetables by substituting the noodles for zucchini noodles. Likewise, you could use lean ground turkey or beans as your protein source instead of ground beef. Fill the sauce with vegetables and spices like spinach, onions, mushrooms, and fresh garlic.

Tip 89: When grocery shopping, fill your cart with lean meats, fish like salmon and tuna, vegetables (esp. dark leafy greens, fruit (esp. berries), whole grains, probiotic-rich foods (ex: yogurt and kombucha), no sugar added sauces, and fresh herbs and spices.

If meal planning still overwhelms you, no worries. I have a 4-week meal plan completely done for you in chapter 7. Following this meal plan will ensure you are consuming those essential nutrients we have discussed so that you can become a healthier person.

Tip 90: When meal planning, have weekly themes like meatless Mondays, Fish Fridays, or Tuna Tuesdays.

This gives you somewhere to start when you are trying to decide what to cook each week.

Tip 91: Make extra and turn your dinner from the night before into lunch the next day.

When you plan to have leftovers, you get two healthy meals in one.

Guidelines for Snacking

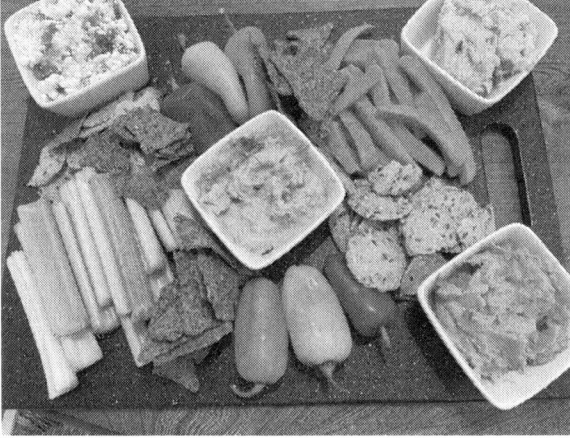

Snacks are a great way to add in foods that may not fit into as many dinner recipes. Below are a few snack tips to keep in mind:

Tip 92: Keep raw vegetables on hand.

If you like to crunch on something throughout the day, then put a few raw veggies into a container and have them available whenever you need a quick snack. You can also munch on these low-calorie, nutrient-dense snacks when you are feeling bored or need a little brain break from work.

Tip 93: Look for packaged snacks that have whole foods listed as the first ingredient.

The first ingredient listed is the dominant ingredient in the package. So, if you see something like whole grains, nuts, seeds, or oats listed as the first ingredient, then you know a whole food is the main ingredient in that packaged snack.

Tip 94: Limit purchasing packages that list trans-fat or added sugar on the label.

As we learned earlier, frequently eating foods with these ingredients increases the risk of a multitude of conditions.

Tip 95: Look for packaged snacks with simple whole food ingredients.

Although it is not always the case, when a label has a long list of unrecognizable ingredients, they may be extra processed.

Tip 96: Look for helpful nutrients in the packaged snack.

Does the snack contain omega-3s, antioxidants, probiotics, or fiber? Then that may be a great snack addition for you.

Review of Chapter 5

- Eat mostly plant-based.
- Eat whole grains 2 to 3 times a day
- Eat vegetables at every meal.
- Eat fruit once a day.
- Eat nuts and seeds about five times a week.
- Eat beans and legumes about four times a week.
- Eat fish two times a week.
- Eat probiotics 4 to 5 times a week.

Chapter 6: Which Supplements Can I Use to Become a Healthier Person?

Although food has the most impact on our health, supplements may provide some benefits as well. For this chapter, we will look at some of the most well-researched supplements and their benefits. But remember, before you take supplements, you should talk with your doctor about any possible interactions with medications or medical conditions. Some supplements can also be toxic when taken in excess, which is another reason to talk with your doctor or dietitian first.

Below is a List of Common Supplements and Their Possible Benefits, Based on Current Research:

Creatine

Creatine has been well studied for its possible benefits to the athlete, and most research shows that creatine does appear to improve athletic performance and strength (60, 88).

Ashwagandha

Tip 97: Instead of unwinding with a less healthy alcoholic drink, try unwinding with a supplement or drink that contains Lemon Balm or Ashwagandha. You can also try sipping on a calming green tea or chamomile tea with a drop of CBD.

According to a systemic review, Ashwagandha may improve VO2 Max in athletes. In addition, some studies also show Ashwagandha may improve symptoms of stress, anxiety, and bipolar disorder (72, 102).

Lemon Balm

Evidence suggests that Lemon Balm may help reduce anxiety symptoms (113).

Non-THC Containing CBD

Tip 98: CBD may be helpful to take before a stressful presentation or public speaking event.

Both animal and human trials have shown CBD may help reduce anxiety and depression. According to a double-blinded, placebo-controlled study on humans, CBD may reduce anxiety and stress related to public speaking. In addition, a mice study indicated that CBD might have anti-depressant properties.

Note: Check the CBD laws in your state before using CBD.

Collagen

Taking collagen as a supplement may increase skin elasticity and hydration and help the skin look younger (22).

Ginger

Tip 99: Ginger and Tart Cherry Juice may help with muscle soreness, so consider consuming these before you go to bed after an intense workout.

In a randomized placebo-controlled trial, ginger appeared to reduce muscle pain from exercise by 25% (15).

Rhodiola Rosea

Some research suggests Rhodiola may improve athletic performance and endurance (10, 99).

According to some early research, Rhodiola may also improve mood disorders like anxiety, depression, and feelings of stress (8).

Holy Basil

According to extensive research, including a systemic review of 24 studies, Holy Basil may reduce symptoms of stress (49, 111).

Vitamin C

Although vitamin C supplements don't seem to prevent a cold in the general population, they may help prevent colds in endurance athletes. In addition, vitamin C supplements may slightly shorten the duration of colds in both athletes and the general population (42, 109).

Omega-3

Tip 100: If you find it hard to get enough omega-3 from food, consider taking a multi-vitamin that contains DHA Omega-3.

We know that according to both animal and human studies, omega-3 helps promote brain function, prevent cognitive decline, and support memory, but one study looked at the benefits of DHA omega-3 on specifically athletes. In this placebo-controlled study, young female soccer players had a better reaction time when they consumed DHA omega-3 (32, 35, 93). And according to a few animal and human studies, omega-3 supplements may help in the recovery of Traumatic Brain Injury (24, 41).

Elderberry

Tip 101: During the fall and winter months, when flu and colds are common, you may want to consider taking a supplement containing a combination of elderberry, zinc, Vitamin D3, and Vitamin C.

Although elderberry doesn't seem to prevent the flu, substantial evidence shows that elderberry may shorten the duration of the flu by 56% (2-4 days) when taken within 48 hours of the first signs of the flu. Flu symptoms also seem to be less severe if you are taking elderberry (33).

Zinc

Zinc supplements may prevent colds and/or reduce the duration and severity, according to 15 studies (33).

Review of Chapter 6

- Supplements that may help with mood are Ashwagandha, CBD, Lemon Balm, Rhodiola, and Holy Basil.
- Vitamin C, Elderberry, and Zinc supplements support the immune system.
- Ginger, creatine, Ashwagandha, and Rhodiola may help improve athletic performance. Vitamin C may help support the immune system in endurance athletes.
- Omega-3 supplements may promote cognitive function.
- Collagen may be a useful anti-aging skin supplement.

Chapter 7: Get the "Right" Foods and Become a Healthier Person with This 4-Week Meal Plan

If you finish reading this, and you think to yourself, "I still need a little extra help." No worries. I have provided a meal plan and recipes for you. If you follow this meal plan, you can confidently know you are consuming plenty of the amazing nutrients we talked about throughout this book. This meal plan is also conducive to weight loss because these meals are:

- Low in Calories
- High in Nutrients
- High in Filling Fiber
- High in Protein

If you need to eat more calories, simply eat more at each meal, add a vegetable side, or add a snack to your day. You can look up your general calorie range below, but you will often find when you listen to your body's hunger cues, you will eat the amount of food that is right for you. If you eat slowly and follow the mindful eating technique from Chapter 4, you will notice you are full and satisfied with smaller portions than if you ate quickly and mindlessly.

General Calorie Guidelines:

- Lightly Active Female between the heights of 5'1"-5'2": Calories per day: 1200
- Lightly Active Female between the heights of 5'3"-5'5": Calories per day: 1300-1400
- Lightly Active Female between the heights of 5'6"-5'9": Calories per day: 1500-1700
- Lightly Active Female between the heights of 6': Calories per day: 1800

- Lightly Active Males between the heights of 5'3"-5'4": Calories per day: 1400-1500
- Lightly Active Males between the heights of 5'5"-5'7": Calories per day: 1600-1700

4-Week Meal Plan

I included a calorie range for each meal and day of this meal plan. The calorie range is an approximation and will vary greatly. The calories will vary based on brands and even slight differences in cooking methods. Every time we cook, our meals come out slightly different. We may use slightly more vegetables or oil, or maybe we added a little more ground chicken than the recommended pound. Many of the meals are "Build Your Own," meaning you will build a slightly different meal with different calorie ranges each day. Remember, if you need more calories, simply eat a larger portion at meals or add one or two snacks during your day. Most people don't need less than 1600, but if you are smaller in stature and do not get much physical activity in your day, you may need less than 1600 calories.

I was very intentional when deciding which recipes and meals to include each day and each week. I wanted to make sure each week contained entirely plant-based meals, animal-based protein meals, and fish meals. I included different herbs and spices in a variety of recipes because fresh herbs and spices are tremendously beneficial to our health. I also made sure to include a variety of vegetables and fruit, and I incorporated those powerhouse berries and dark leafy greens frequently. I also provided a combination of low-calorie meals with meals that were slightly higher in calories and high in nutrients. Since both lower and moderate calorie meals are included on the same days, the calories balance out.

Most of these meal plans are under 1,600 calories, so for most, you will need to add a vegetable side and some snacks throughout the day.

A Note on the Breakfast and Lunch Meals

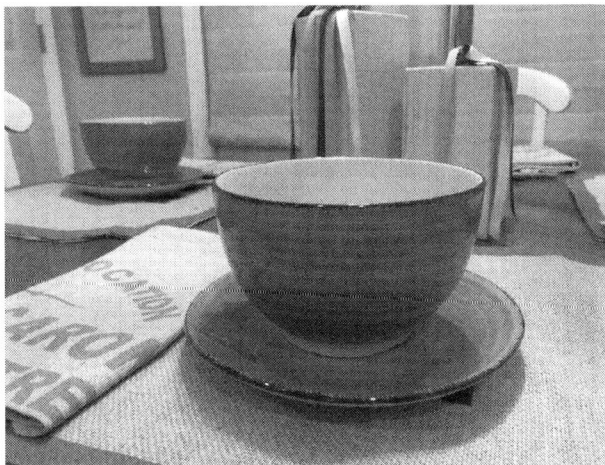

You will notice that for breakfast and lunch, I rotate between some of the same few meals. This is because these meals provide a huge amount of variety within themselves. In addition, many of these meals are "Build Your Own," so you can build something different each day. For example, say Monday, you decide to make a turkey sandwich for your "Build Your Own Sandwich" meal, but on Thursday, you decide to make a hummus sandwich when you "Build Your Own Sandwich." Or maybe one day you have tuna salad on a bed of leafy greens for your "Build Your Own Salad," but then a few days later, you have a salad topped with salsa and pre-packaged grilled chicken. The "Build Your Own" recipes provide a list of ingredients to pick and choose from, so you can easily find new meals to eat.

Cooking Efficiently Tips

Sometimes our lives get busy, and some nights we just don't have time to make a recipe. However, you can do a few things to make cooking these recipes easier.

1. Do a little Sunday prep work. Look through your recipes for the week. Spend some time chopping your vegetables and even cooking your meat on Sunday. You can make your cloud bread beforehand as well.
2. Buy pre-cooked or pre-chopped vegetables. Although these recipes are usually healthier than store-bought, you can still use store-bought versions for some of these recipes if you find yourself in a time crunch. Some store-bought alternatives you can use are store-bought guacamole, hummus, pre-cooked grilled chicken, rotisserie chicken, and Pico De Gallo.
3. You can also use quick versions, like minute brown rice or instant quinoa. Just follow the package directions unless I already use the instant version in the recipe.
4. You can double the recipe and eat it for two nights or eat the leftovers for lunch the next day.
5. Many of the recipes require no cooking. Choose these options when you just don't have time to cook. You can even use recipes like "Build Your Own Salad" for dinner on busy nights.

Week 1

Day 1 (1,685 calories):

Breakfast: 1 cup of "Build Your Own Parfait" (150-200 calories)

Lunch: 1 1/2 cup of "Classic Hummus Dip" with 1 cup of raw carrot and celery sticks and ½ cup whole-grain crackers. (I like the Mary's Gone Crackers Brand) (645 calories)

Dinner: 1 1/2 cup of "Pesto Salmon with Zoodles" (840 calories)

Day 2: (1,205-1,705 calories)

Breakfast: 8 ounces of "Chocolate Blueberry Oat Milk Smoothie" (415 calories)

Lunch: 2 cups of "Build Your Own Salad" (300-800 calories)

Dinner: 1 Cup of "Chicken Tikka Masala over Yellow Rice" (490 calories)

Day 3 (900-1,550 calories):

Breakfast: 1 cup of "Build Your Own Trail Mix" (400-550 calories)

Lunch: 1 "Build Your Own Sandwich" (300-800 calories)

Dinner: 2 cups of "Pico De Gallo Cauliflower Rice Bowl" (200 calories)

Day 4 (1,400 calories):

Breakfast: 3 "Build Your Own Energy Protein Ball" (300-400 calories)

Lunch: 11/2 cup of "Chicken Salad Dip" with 1 cup of raw carrot and celery sticks and 1 cup whole-grain crackers. (I like the Mary's Gone Crackers Brand) (500 calories)

Dinner: 4 "Ginger Soy Lettuce Wraps" (500 calories)

Day 5 (850-1,400 calories):

Breakfast: 1 cup of "Build Your Own Parfait" (150-200 calories)

Lunch: 2 cups of "Build Your Own Salad" (300-800 calories)

Dinner: 2 cups of "Spicy Quinoa with Vegetables" (400 calories)

Day 6 (1,200-1,800 calories):

Breakfast: 3 "Build Your Own Energy Protein Ball" (300-400 calories)

Lunch: 1 "Build Your Own Sandwich" (300-800 calories)

Dinner: 2 cups of "Breakfast Bowl for Dinner" (600 calories)

Day 7 (1,245 calories):

Breakfast: 8 ounces of "Chocolate Blueberry Oat Milk Smoothie" (415 calories)

Lunch: 1 cup "Layered Taco Dip" with whole-grain tortilla chips (400 calories)

Dinner: 1 "Salmon Cloud Bread Taco" (430 calories)

Week 2

Day 1 (1,000-1,550 calories):

Breakfast: 1 cup of "Build Your Own Trail Mix" (400-550 calories)

Lunch: 2 cups of "Build Your Own Salad" (300-800 calories)

Dinner: 2 cups "Tangy Konjac Noodles with Vegetables" (200 calories)

Day 2 (850-1,400 calories):

Breakfast: 1 Cup of "Build your Own Yogurt Parfait" (150-200 calories)

Lunch: 1 "Build your Own Sandwich" (300-800 calories)

Dinner: 1 "Supreme Cloud Bread Pizza" (400 calories)

Day 3 (1,200-1,300 calories):

Breakfast: 3 "Build Your Own Energy Protein Ball" (300-400 calories)

Lunch: 1 cup of "Black-Eyed Peas Dip" with 1 cup of raw carrot and celery sticks and ½ cup whole grain (300 calories)

Dinner: 1 cup "Chickpeas and Turmeric over Yellow Rice" (600 calories)

Day 4 (1,115-1,615 calories):

Breakfast: 8 ounces of "Chocolate Blueberry Oat Milk Smoothie" (415 calories)

Lunch: 2 cups of "Build your Own Salad" (300-800 calories)

Dinner: 1 cup of "Taco Pasta" (400 calories)

Day 5 (1,100-1,250 calories):

Breakfast: 1 cup of "Build Your Own Trail Mix" (400-550 calories)

Lunch: "Turkey Jerky Spread" with 1 cup of raw carrot and celery sticks and ½ cup whole grain (400 calories)

Dinner: 1 "Chickpea Lettuce Wrap" (300 calories)

Day 6 (800-1,400 calories):

Breakfast: 3 "Build Your Own Energy Protein Balls" (300-400 calories)

Lunch: 1 "Build Your Own Sandwich" (300-800 calories)

Dinner: 1 "Vegetable Cloud Bread Pizza" (200 calories)

Day 7 (950-1,500 calories):

Breakfast: 1 cup of "Build your Own Yogurt Parfait" (150-200 calories)

Lunch: 2 cups of "Build Your Own Salad (300-800 calories)

Dinner: 1 cup "Chicken Lo Mein" (500 calories)

Week 3

Day 1 (900-1,500 calories):

Breakfast: 3 "Build Your Own Energy Protein Balls" (300-400 calories)

Lunch: 1 Build Your Own Sandwich (300-800 calories)

Dinner: 1 cup of "Pesto Pasta" (300 calories)

Day 2 (915 calories):

Breakfast: 8 ounces of "Chocolate Blueberry Oat Milk Smoothie" (415 calories)

Lunch: "Creamy Avocado Ranch Dip" with 1 cup of raw carrot and celery sticks and 1 cup whole grain (300 calories)

Dinner: 2 cups "Mushroom Soup" (200 calories)

Day 3 (750-1,300 calories):

Breakfast: 1 cup of "Build your Own Yogurt Parfait" (150-200 calories)

Lunch: 2 cups of "Build Your Own Salad (300-800 calories)

Dinner: 1 cup "Turkey Chili" (300 calories)

Day 4 (1,050-1,700 calories):

Breakfast: 1 cup of "Build Your Own Trail Mix" (400-550 calories)

Lunch:1 "Build Your Own Sandwich" (300-800 calories)

Dinner: 1 "Pesto Pizza Tortilla" (350 calories)

Day 5 (1,100-1,200 calories):

Breakfast: 3 "Build Your Own Energy Protein Balls" (300-400 calories)

Lunch: "Classic Guac Dip" with 1 cup of raw carrot and celery sticks and ½ cup whole grain (300 calories)

Dinner: 2 "Fish Tacos" (500 calories)

Day 6 (1,115-1,615 calories):

Breakfast: 8 ounces of "Chocolate Blueberry Oat Milk Smoothie" (415 calories)

Lunch: 2 cups of "Build Your Own Salad" (300-800 calories)

Dinner: 1 slice of "Palmini Lasagna" (400 calories)

Day 7:

Breakfast: 1 cup of "Build your Own Yogurt Parfait" (150-200 calories)

Lunch: 1 "Build Your Own Sandwich" (300-800 calories)

Dinner: 1 "Pesto Grilled Cheese Sandwich on Wheat Bread" (400 calories)

Week 4

Day 1 (1,000-1,650 calories):

Breakfast: 1 cup of "Build Your Own Trail Mix" (400-550 calories)

Lunch: 2 cups of "Build Your Own Salad" (300-800 calories)

Dinner: 1 cup of "Taco Chili" (300 calories)

Day 2 (900-1,500 calories):

Breakfast: 3 "Build Your Own Energy Protein Balls" (300-400 calories)

Lunch: 1 "Build Your Own Sandwich" (300-800 calories)

Dinner: 1 cup of "Comfort Baked Spaghetti" (300 calories)

Day 3 (1,115 calories):

Breakfast: 8 ounces of "Chocolate Blueberry Oat Milk Smoothie" (415 calories)

Lunch: 1 cup of "Buffalo Ranch Chicken Dip" with 1 cup of raw carrot and celery sticks and ½ cup whole grain (300 calories)

Dinner: 1 Italian Meatball Cloud Bread Sandwich" (400 calories)

Day 4 (750-1,300 calories):

Breakfast: 1 cup of "Build your Own Yogurt Parfait" (150-200 calories)

Lunch: 2 cups of "Build Your Own Salad" (300-800 calories)

Dinner: 2 cups "Tangy Konjac Noodles with Vegetables" (300 calories)

Day 5 (1,000-1,650 calories):

Breakfast: 1 cup of "Build Your Own Trail Mix" (400-550 calories)

Lunch: 1 "Build Your Own Sandwich" (300-800 calories)

Dinner: 2 cups "Sweet and Sour Meatballs over Cauliflower Rice" (300 calories)

Day 6 (900-1,500 calories):

Breakfast: 3 "Build Your Own Energy Protein Balls" (300-400 calories)

Lunch: 2 cups of "Build Your Own Salad" (300-800 calories)

Dinner: 1 "Open-Faced BBQ Chicken Sandwich" (300 calories)

Day 7 (1,115-1,615 calories):

Breakfast: 8 ounces of "Chocolate Blueberry Oat Milk Smoothie" (415 calories)

Lunch: 1 "Build Your Own Sandwich" (300-800 calories)

Dinner: 1 "Greek Yogurt Mayo Open-Faced Turkey Sandwich" (400 calories)

Bonus Day (750-1,300 calories):

Breakfast: 1 cup of "Build your Own Yogurt Parfait" (150-200 calories)

Lunch: 2 cups of "Build Your Own Salad" (300-800 calories)

Dinner: 1 cup of "Black Bean Soup" (300 calories)

Healthy Snack Ideas:

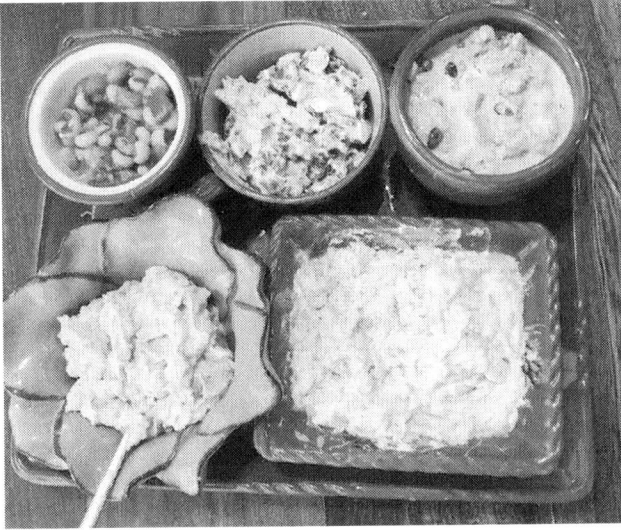

- Black-eyed Pea Dip with Crackers (Recipe in Chapter 8)
- Jerky Dip with crackers (Recipe in Chapter 8)
- Build Your Own Energy Balls (Recipe in Chapter 8)
- Black Bean Hummus (Recipe in Chapter 8)
- Classic Hummus (Recipe in Chapter 8)
- Pico De Gallo and chips (Recipe in Chapter 8)
- Guacamole and chips or vegetable sticks (Recipe in Chapter 8)
- Yogurt Avocado Ranch and vegetable sticks (Recipe in Chapter 8)
- Chips and salsa
- Build your own trail mix (Recipe in Chapter 8)
- Nutrition Bar
- Build your own Yogurt Parfait (Recipe in Chapter 8)
- A piece of fruit (apple, orange, pear)
- A cup of fruit (pineapple chunks, blueberries, grapes, strawberries)
- Cloud bread with light cream cheese and fruit topping (Recipe in Chapter 8)

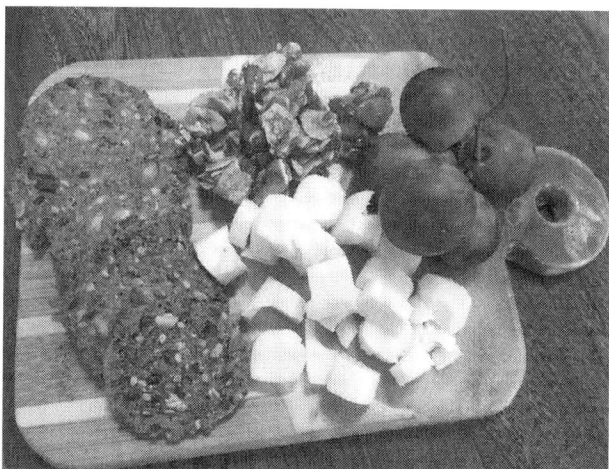

Chapter 8: Meal Plan Recipes

Breakfast Recipes

You will notice I made the recipes easy and quick for breakfast, and I did this for a reason. Mornings are often hectic for many, and we just don't have time to cook huge meals. All of these recipes require absolutely no cooking and can be eaten for several days. For efficiency, you can choose to eat the same breakfast for multiple days in a row if you would like. For example, if you made the Chocolate Blueberry Oat Milk Smoothie, you may decide to drink the smoothie every day until you run out of smoothies. After you run out of smoothies, you might decide to make the "Build Your Own Energy Protein Balls" and eat those every day until you finish the whole batch. Or, if you like variety, you can eat your breakfast in the order suggested in the meal plan. All the recipes are super nourishing, so it doesn't matter what order you eat them.

Build Your Own Yogurt Parfait (Pick and Choose from the Ingredients Below)

Berries, nuts, seeds, and yogurt are sometimes tricky to get into your meal plan. They don't always fit into a savory meal so well, but they are so important for our health. These parfaits are a perfect way to ensure you are getting these vital ingredients into your everyday meals. You can also sneak in a few other superstar ingredients like collagen powder and matcha green tea powder. Cinnamon is an important spice that goes well in sweet recipes. Cinnamon acts as an antioxidant and is a good source of calcium, fiber, iron, and manganese.

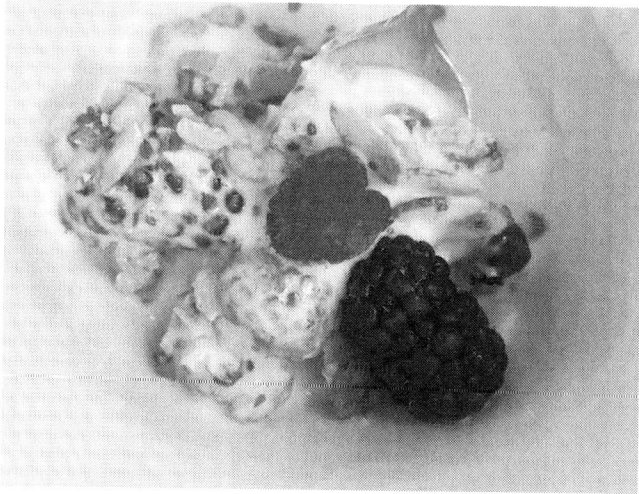

Servings: 1

Ingredients:

- 1/4 cup of nuts or seeds (Pick one: walnuts, pistachios, pecans, almonds, or pumpkin seeds, sunflower seeds)
- 1/4 cup berries (Pick one: blueberries, blackberries raspberries, acai berries, strawberries)
- 1 cup light vanilla Greek yogurt with probiotics
- 1/4 teaspoon of your favorite flavoring (Pick one: Cinnamon, vanilla extract, almond extract)
- Optional add-ins: (Pick one: 1/4 teaspoon collagen powder, 1/4 teaspoon Matcha green tea extract)

Instructions:

To make this recipe, simply combine all the ingredients of your choice and enjoy! That is it! Super simple and super nourishing!

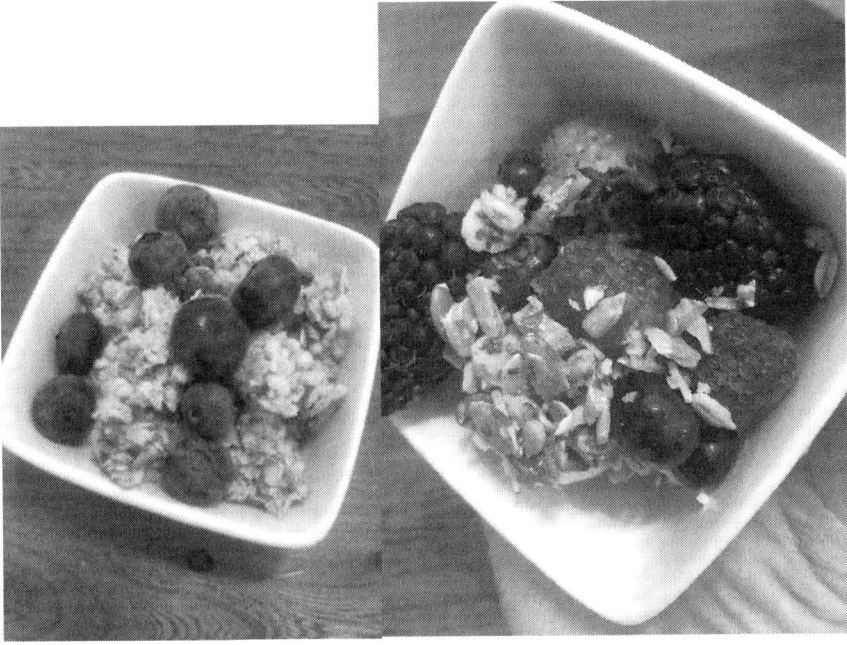

Chocolate Blueberry Oat Milk Smoothie

This is another recipe that packs in a lot of nourishment at once. Drink this for breakfast, and you will have already consumed antioxidants, ALA omega-3s, vitamins, and minerals, and your day has just begun. Even if the rest of your day gets super hectic and you couldn't eat as many nourishing foods as you would have liked, you can take comfort in knowing you were able to pack in a lot of helpful nutrients in the morning.

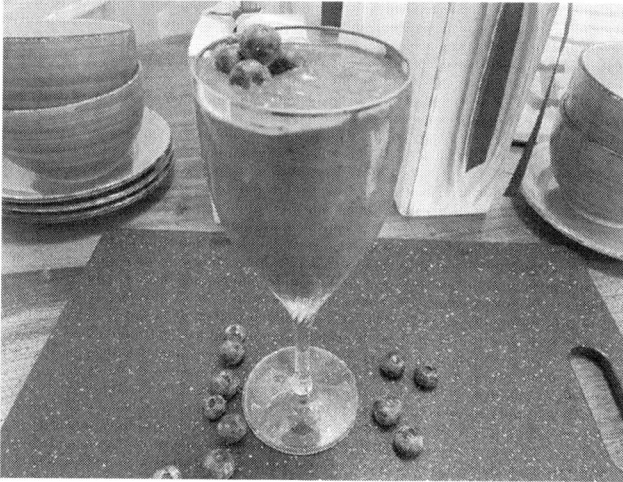

Servings: 5

Ingredients:

- 1/2 cup dark chocolate chips
- 1/4 cup ground flaxseed powder or chia seed
- 1/2 cup Greek yogurt
- 1/2 cup blueberries
- 1/4 cup
- 1/4 cup matcha green tea powder or collagen powder
- 1 Tablespoon almond extract
- 1/2 cup dates
- 2 cup regular or vanilla oat milk

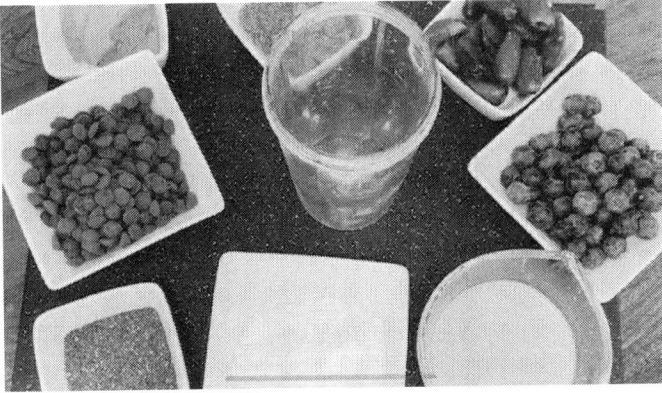

Instructions:

1. Add all the ingredients into a large blender.
2. Blend until the ingredients are well blended and smooth.
3. Chill in the refrigerator until you are ready to enjoy your drink.

Build Your Own Trail Mix (Pick and Choose from the Ingredients Below)

This might be one of the easiest breakfast recipes you will ever make. It even works great for a "hurry we are going to be late for school, grab it, let's go" breakfast. It requires no cooking, cutting, or even prepping. You just combine a bunch of crunchy, savory, and sweet, healthy packaged treats, and it's done!

I didn't include amounts for this recipe because you can decide to add as little or as much of each ingredient as you want. A serving size would be about 1 cup of trail mix.

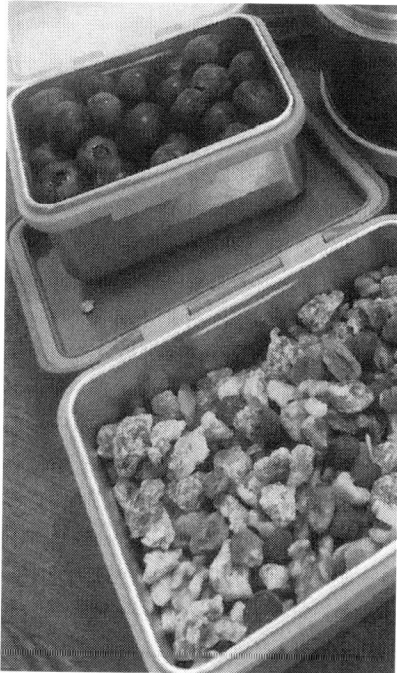

Serving size: 1 cup

Ingredients:

- **Something Sweet (Pick 2 or 3 from the choices below):**
    - Dried fruit (dried cranberries, bananas, coconut, apples, apricots, pineapples)
    - Fresh berries (blueberries, blackberries, raspberries, acai berries, strawberries)
    - Raisins
    - Dark chocolate chips
    - Dark chocolate almonds
    - Packaged granola clusters

- **Add Something Savory (Pick 2 or 3 from the choices below):**
- Whole Grain Chex cereal
- Packaged nut clusters
- Popcorn
- No Nitrate/Nitrite Added Free-Range Turkey jerky or Grass-fed beef jerky
- Nuts and Seeds (Almonds, walnuts, cashews, pistachios, peanuts, pumpkin seeds)
- Roasted chickpeas
- Edamame beans

Instructions:

- Make this trail mix your own. Pick and choose your favorite ingredients and mix them together.
- And done! So simple! And no cooking required! Talk about a quick on-the-go breakfast!

Build Your Own Energy Protein Ball (Pick and Choose from the Ingredients Below)

My mornings are chaotic, and as you can see, I like to keep breakfast simple. This recipe requires no cooking and can be made ahead of time. Since this recipe makes ten balls, you can eat on this recipe for days unless your family eats them all.

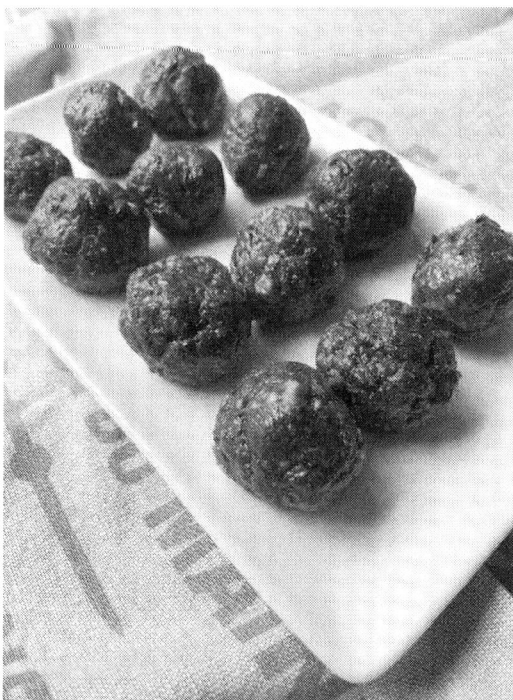

Servings: 10 (Makes about 10 balls)

Basic Ingredients (Use this in every recipe):

- 1 1/2 cup rolled oats or granola
- 1/2 cup any nut or seed butter (peanut butter, almond butter, mixed nut butter, hazelnut butter, macadamia nut butter, pumpkin seed butter, hemp seed butter, mixed seed butter, etc.)

98

Other Ingredients (Pick and Choose from Below):

- Dark chocolate chips
- Raisins
- Dried cranberries
- Coconut
- Crumbled nuts and seeds (almonds, walnuts, cashews, pistachios, peanuts, pumpkin seeds)
- Dates, pitted

Add Some Sweetness (Pick and Choose from Below):

- 1/4 teaspoon cinnamon
- 1 teaspoon honey
- 1/4 teaspoon almond extract or vanilla extract

Optional Super Ingredients (Pick and Choose from Below):

- Matcha green tea
- Collagen powder
- Ground flaxseed

Instructions:

- In a large food processor, blend all the ingredients, including whichever optional ingredient you choose. Mix until the ingredients form a dough consistency.
- Roll the dough into bite-size balls.
- Store in the refrigerator until you are ready to eat.

Lunch Recipes

Here is how the lunches work. Just like the breakfast recipes, I made them easy. In addition, I made it easily portable so that you can take them to work. Some of the recipes are for dips and can be used in other recipes and as a snack. For example, the hummus can be eaten with crackers and vegetables for lunch or a snack or added to the "Build Your Own Salad" recipe.

Classic Hummus Dip

Hummus is a perfect plant-based protein dip. It is creamy and full of flavor and nutrients. Chickpeas are a prebiotic and good fiber, folate, vitamin B6, iron, and zinc.

Serves: 6-8

Ingredients:

- 1 can chickpeas
- 1/4 cup tahini
- 1/4 cup extra virgin olive oil
- 2 teaspoons lemon juice
- 1/2 teaspoon minced garlic
- 1/4 teaspoon salt
- 1/2 teaspoon cumin
- 2 Tablespoons water
- 1/4 teaspoon hot sauce (optional)

Instructions:

- Blend all the ingredients together in a food processor until well blended.
- Serve with raw carrots, celery sticks, red, yellow, or orange pepper sticks, and/or whole-grain crackers, or add a scoop to the top of your "Build Your Own Salad" or "Build Your Own Sandwich."

Build Your Own Salad

By building your own salad, you can add variety to your daily lunches. In addition, you can change the ingredients to make your salad feel completely different on a daily basis. For example, add more fruit to make the salad sweet, leave off the animal protein to make the salad plant-based, or add a scoop of chicken salad to make the salad hearty.

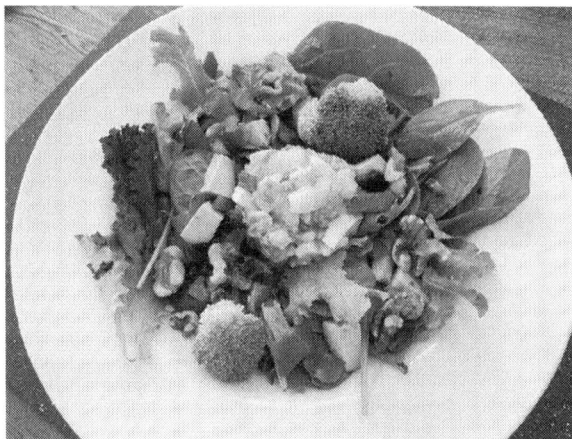

Ingredients:

Basic Ingredients (Use one or more of these in every recipe):

- Lettuce
- Spinach
- Kale
- Spring mix
- Arugula

Add a Protein (Pick one or more):

- Nuts: almonds, walnuts, cashews, mixed nuts, pistachios
- Seeds: sunflower, pumpkin
- Chickpeas

- Boiled eggs
- Black beans
- Chicken Salad (see recipe below)
- Salmon Salad (see recipe below)
- Hummus (see recipe above)
- Tuna Salad (see recipe below)
- Turkey Slices, chopped (look for no nitrite/no nitrate added turkey slices)
- Black-eyed pea dip (see recipe below)
- Canned beans (black beans, kidney beans)
- Edamame
- Buffalo Ranch Chicken Dip (see recipe below)
- Black Bean Hummus (see recipe below)

Add Vegetables (pick one or more):

- Blanched Asparagus (Place asparagus in a colander in the sink. Meanwhile boil water on the stove. Then carefully pour the hot water over the vegetables in the colander.)
- Blanched Brussel Sprouts, halves or shredded (Blanch the same way you would blanch asparagus.)
- Blanched or raw zucchini (I prefer them blanched)
- Blanched or raw squash (I prefer them blanched)
- Broccoli
- Cauliflower
- Tomato slices
- Cherry tomatoes
- Carrots
- Cucumber
- Corn
- Onion, chopped
- Peppers, chopped
- Roasted Red Peppers
- Olives
- Red Cabbage
- Avocado Slices

Optional Dips:

- Salsa
- Avocado Ranch Dip (see recipe below)
- Guacamole (see recipe below)
- Pico De Gallo (see recipe below)

If You Want Something Sweet Add a Little Fruit

- Blueberries
- Grapes
- Strawberries
- Raspberries

Dressing (Pick One):

- Ranch Yogurt Dressing (see recipe below)
- Vinaigrettes
- Asian Dressing
- Dressing made with no sugar added and made with healthy oils like extra virgin olive oil. (brands will note this on the label)

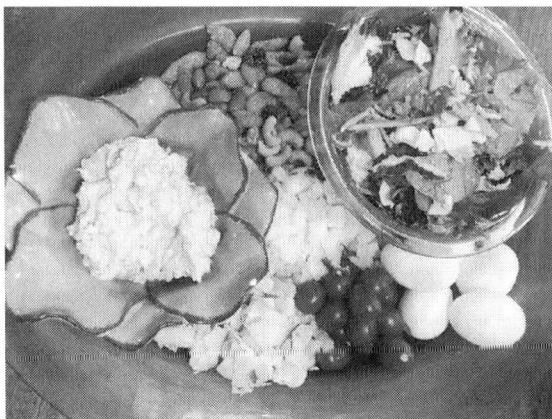

Instructions:

- Add one or a combination of leafy greens onto a plate.
- Add one or more ingredients from the protein list.
- Add one or more ingredients from the vegetable list
- If you would like, add a dip.

- Drizzle with a healthy dressing.
- A serving should equal about 2 cups.

Build Your Own Sandwich

This recipe is similar to the "Build Your Own Salad" recipe because you get to pick and choose what goes in your sandwich every day. You start with deciding what is going to hold your ingredients, then you add a protein, vegetables, and some seasoning and condiments, and you have a delicious and nutritious lunch.

Ingredients:

"Bread" Ingredients (Pick one of These to "Hold" Your Other Ingredients):

- Whole wheat bread (you can use just one piece and make the sandwich open-faced if you would like)
- Lettuce (to make a lettuce wrap)
- Whole-grain tortilla

Add a Protein (Pick one or more):

- Chicken Salad (see recipe)
- Salmon Salad (see recipe)
- Hummus (see recipe)
- Tuna Salad (see recipe)
- Turkey Slices, chopped (look for no nitrite/no nitrate added turkey slices)
- Buffalo Ranch Chicken Dip (see recipe)
- Black Bean Hummus (see recipe)
- Pre-cooked grilled chicken strips
- Pre-packaged frozen black bean burger

Add Vegetables (pick one or more):

- Tomato sliced
- Cucumber
- Onion, sliced
- Lettuce
- Spinach

- Kale
- Spring mix
- Arugula
- Peppers, sliced
- Roasted red peppers
- Olives
- Red cabbage
- Avocado slices

Add a Dip:

- Avocado Ranch Dip (See recipe below)
- Guacamole (see recipe below)

Add a Condiment (Pick One):

- Ranch Yogurt Dressing (see Recipe Below)
- Vinaigrettes
- Oil and vinegar
- Mayo made with extra virgin olive oil
- mustard
- Dressing made with no sugar added and made with healthy oils like extra virgin olive oil. (Brands will note this on the label)
- Hot Sauce

Instructions:

- Pick your "bread."
- Add one or more ingredients from the protein list.
- Add one or more ingredients from the vegetable list
- If you would like, add a dip.
- Spread your favorite condiments on the sandwich.

Chicken Salad Dip

You use canned chicken for this recipe, so you don't need to do any cooking. This chicken salad tastes fantastic on top of whole-grain crackers or added to a sandwich or salad.

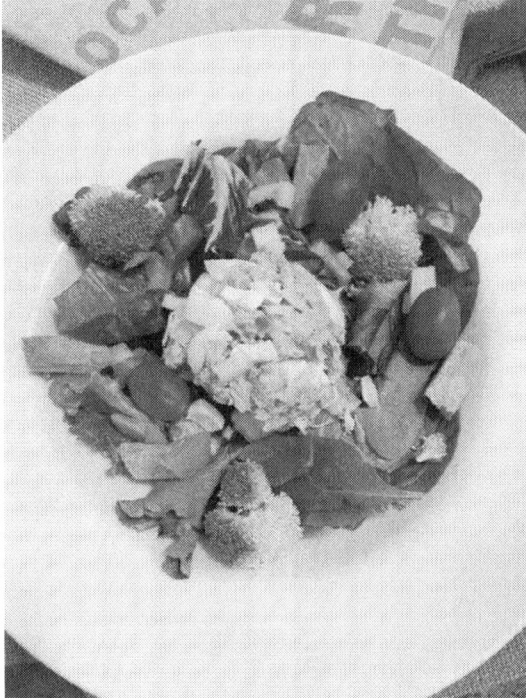

Servings: 4

Ingredients:

- 12.5 oz. canned white meat chicken
- 1 stalk celery, washed and chopped
- 1/4 cup walnuts
- 1/4 cup red grapes, washed and sliced
- 1 teaspoon black pepper
- 1/4 cup plain Greek yogurt
- 1/4 teaspoon salt
- 1 clove garlic, minced
- 1/2 teaspoon extra virgin olive oil

Instructions:

- Mix all the ingredients together in a medium bowl.
- Chill the chicken salad for 30 minutes in the refrigerator before serving.
- Serve with raw carrots, celery sticks, red, yellow, or orange pepper sticks, and/or whole-grain crackers, or add a scoop to the top of your "Build Your Own Salad" or "Build your Own Sandwich."

Layered Taco Dip

Layers of nutritional goodness, this layered Taco Dip is perfect for lunch, a snack, or as an appetizer. The beans add fiber and protein, and the yogurt adds probiotics. By using spinach leaves instead of lettuce leaves, you are including those all-important dark leafy greens.

Servings: 4-6

Ingredients:

- 8 oz. jar of salsa
- 1 cup yogurt
- 1 cup canned refried beans
- 1 cup cheddar cheese
- 1 tomato, chopped
- 1 cup shredded spinach
- 2 green onions, chopped
- 1 cup cilantro leaves
- 1/2 cup guacamole (see recipe below)

Instructions:

- Mix the salsa and yogurt together in a medium bowl.
- In a medium casserole dish, layer the ingredients in the following order: refried beans, salsa-yogurt mixture, cheese, spinach leaves, tomato, scallions, and cilantro.
- Top with a dollop of guacamole.
- Garnish with a few scallions and cilantro
- Cover and chill the dip in the refrigerator for 45 minutes.
- Serve with whole-grain tortilla chips.

Black-eyed Pea Dip

The black-eyed peas are a great source of plant-based protein, and the vegetables provide plenty of vitamins and minerals. Add this dip to your favorite whole-grain cracker, and you get a quick yet complete meal!

Ingredients:

- 15 oz. can black-eyed peas
- 1 can corn
- 1 tomato, diced
- 1 onion, diced
- 8 oz. Italian vinaigrette
- 1 teaspoon jalapenos, diced
- 1 Tablespoon cilantro

Instructions:

- Combine all the ingredients in a medium bowl. Stir until the ingredients are well mixed together.
- Serve with whole-grain tortillas, chips, or crackers.

Turkey Jerky Spread

This Turkey Jerky Spread provides a creative way to get in more probiotics. When choosing your jerky, look for no nitrate/nitrite added free-range turkey jerky.

Servings: 4-6

Ingredients:

- 1 cup Greek yogurt
- 3 oz bags of free-range, no nitrate/nitrite added turkey jerky (broken up into small pieces)
- 1 tomato, diced
- 3 green onions, diced
- 1 teaspoon garlic, minced
- 2 teaspoons extra virgin olive oil
- 1 teaspoon black pepper

Instructions:

- Break the jerky into small pieces.
- Combine all the ingredients together in a small bowl.
- Refrigerate the spread for about 30 minutes.
- Serve cold with whole-grain crackers or tortilla chips.

Creamy Avocado Ranch Dip

This dip is a hit when I bring it to parties. It's so creamy and savory. It's so good that the party guests never even think about how healthy this dip is. The avocados are a good source of healthy fats, and the Greek yogurt is a good source of gut-healthy probiotics.

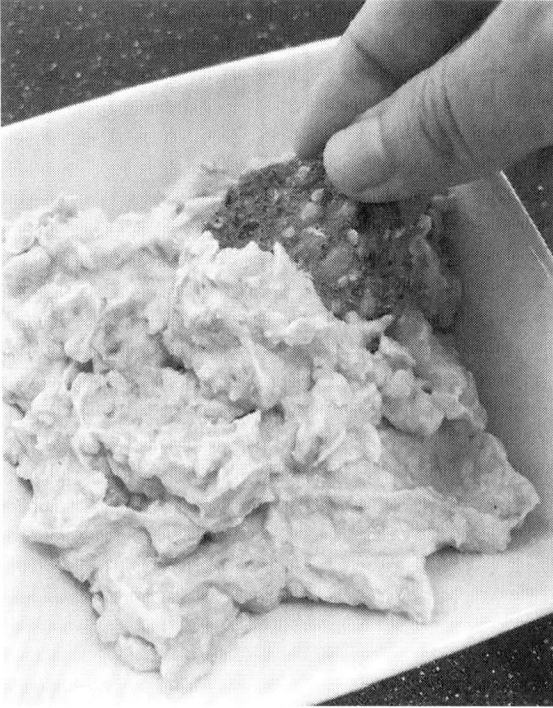

Servings: 4-5

Ingredients:

- 2 avocados, peeled and pitted
- 1/3 cup Greek yogurt, plain
- 1 teaspoon lime or lemon juice
- 2 teaspoons ranch powder
- 1 clove garlic, minced

Instructions:

- Combine all the ingredients in a medium bowl.
- Stir and smash the ingredients with a fork or pestle until they are mixed well.
- Serve with whole-grain chips, crackers, or crispy raw vegetables.

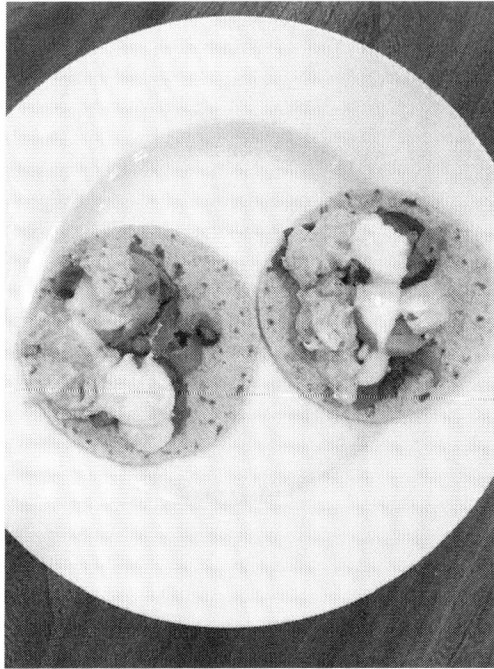

*Ranch Guacamole tastes fantastic on a variety of dishes. Here is Ranch Guacamole on top of vegetable tacos.

Classic Guacamole Dip

Nothing is quite like a delicious bowl of classic guacamole. Of course, you can always purchase an already-made version at the store, but it is never as good as fresh guacamole.

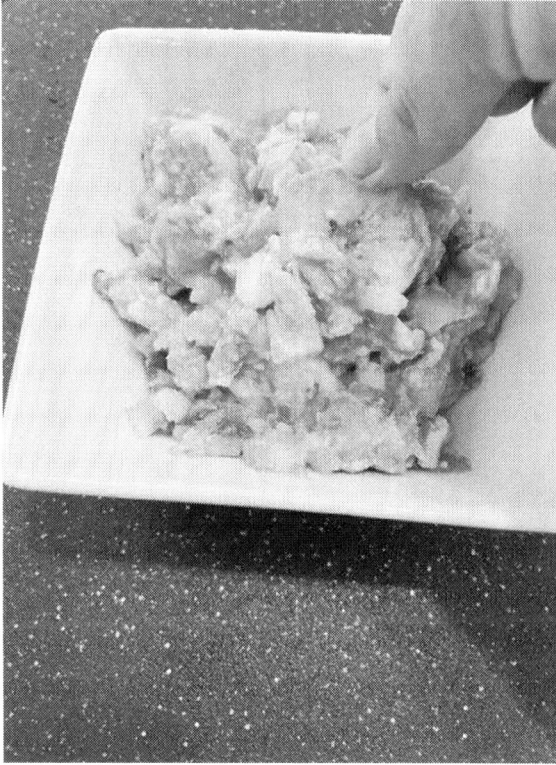

Servings: 6

Ingredients:

- 4 avocados, peeled and pitted
- 2 large tomatoes, diced
- 1/2 cup cilantro
- 1 medium jalapeno, diced
- 1/2 white onion, diced
- 1/2 teaspoon salt
- 4 cloves garlic, minced

- 1/2 cup lime juice

Instructions:

1. Combine all the ingredients in a large bowl. Mash and stir the ingredients together with a fork or pestle until the avocado is smashed to your liking.
2. Serve immediately. Guacamole is best when it's fresh.
3. Serve with whole-grain tortilla chips or crackers.

Buffalo Ranch Chicken Dip

This is another healthy recipe people go nuts for when I bring it to a party. Greek yogurt provides probiotics, and the chicken and nutritional yeast provide the protein. Did you know that nutritional yeast is a plant-based complete protein? This means that nutritional yeast contains all the essential amino acids. In addition, nutritional yeast also contains antioxidants, vitamin B12, and Beta Glucan.

Servings: 8

Ingredients:

- 12.5 ounces canned white meat chicken, drained
- 1/4 cup plain Greek yogurt
- 1/4 cup powdered ranch seasoning
- 4 ounces light cream cheese, softened at room temperature
- 1 cup hot sauce
- 1/4 cup nutritional yeast (this gives the dip a cheesy flavor)

Instructions:

1. Combine and stir all the ingredients in a medium mixing bowl.

2. Cover the bowl with foil and set the bowl in the refrigerator for at least 45 minutes.

3. When you are ready to eat, you can either eat the dip cold or heat it in the microwave for approximately 1 minute or until it is warm.

4. Serve with whole-grain chips or crackers.

Salmon Salad

These next few recipes are for you to add to your "Build Your Own Salad" and "Build Your Own Sandwich" recipes. This Salmon Salad recipe provides an easy way to incorporate DHA Omega-3s into your diet. It's made with canned salmon, so you don't need to cook it.

Servings: 1

Ingredients:

- 1/2 cup wild-caught salmon, canned
- 1 boiled egg, chopped
- 1 Tablespoon dill relish
- 1/2 cup red onion, chopped
- 1/4 teaspoon salt
- 1/4 teaspoon black pepper
- 1 teaspoon lemon juice

Instructions:

- Combine and stir all the ingredients in a small bowl.
- Cover and chill the salmon salad in the refrigerator for about 30 minutes.
- Serve on top of a salad or in a sandwich.

Tuna Salad

I have two Tuna Salad recipes in this book. They are very similar, and the main difference is one contains probiotic-rich Greek yogurt, and one does not. However, both are great sources of DHA Omega-3-rich cold-water fish.

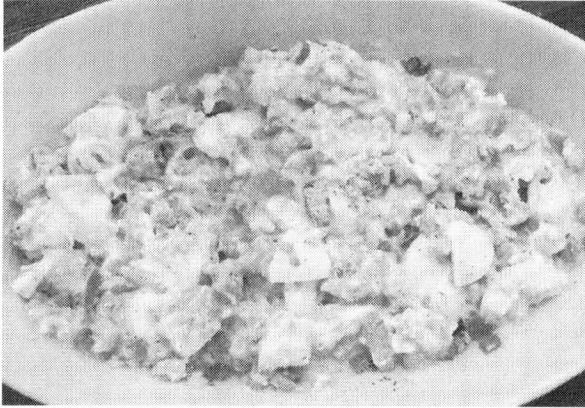

Servings: 1

Ingredients:

- 2.6 oz. wild-caught canned tuna (1/2 cup)
- 1 boiled egg, chopped
- 1 Tablespoon dill relish
- 1/2 cup red onion, chopped
- 1/4 teaspoon salt
- 1/4 teaspoon black pepper
- 1 teaspoon lemon juice

Instructions:

- Combine and stir all the ingredients.
- Cover the bowl with foil and chill in the refrigerator for about 30 minutes.

- Serve on a bed of greens in the "Build Your Own Salad" recipe or as part of a sandwich in the "Build Your Own Sandwich" recipe.

Greek Yogurt Tuna Salad

Servings: 1

Ingredients:

- 2.6 oz. wild-caught canned tuna
- 1/4 cup Greek yogurt
- 2 cloves garlic, minced
- 1 boiled egg, chopped
- 1 Tablespoon dill relish
- 1/2 cup red onion, chopped
- 1/4 teaspoon salt
- 1/4 teaspoon black pepper
- 1 teaspoon lemon juice

Instructions:

- Combine and stir all the ingredients.
- Cover the bowl with foil and chill in the refrigerator for about 30 minutes.
- Serve on a bed of greens in the "Build Your Own Salad" recipe or as part of a sandwich in the "Build Your Own Sandwich" Recipe.

Black Bean Hummus

This plant-based Black Bean Hummus works great as a dip with chips and crackers, as part of a sandwich, or as a topping for a salad.

Servings: 6-8

Ingredients:

- 15 oz. canned black beans
- 1/4 cup ***tahini***
- 1/2 cup extra virgin olive oil
- 2 teaspoons lemon juice
- 3 cloves garlic, minced
- 1/4 teaspoon salt
- 1/2 teaspoon cumin
- 1/2 teaspoon paprika
- 1/4 teaspoon cayenne pepper
- 2 Tablespoons water

Instructions:

- Combine and stir all the ingredients and done!
- Serve with whole grain chips, tortillas, or raw vegetables or on a bed of greens in the "Build Your Own Salad" recipe or as part of a sandwich in the "Build Your Own Sandwich" recipe.

Greek Yogurt Ranch Dressing

This dressing was mentioned as a dressing option for the "Build Your Own Salad" recipe. You can also use it as a spread in the "Build Your Own Sandwich" recipe. The star ingredient in this recipe is the probiotic-rich Greek yogurt.

Ingredients:

- 3/4 cup Greek yogurt
- 1 Tablespoon fresh lemon
- 1 avocado, peeled and mashed
- 1 teaspoon white vinegar
- 1 teaspoon parsley
- 1/2 teaspoon dill

- 3 cloves garlic, minced
- 1 teaspoon onion powder
- 1 teaspoon chives
- 1/2 teaspoon black pepper
- 1/4 teaspoon sea salt

Instructions:

- Using a food processor, blend all ingredients until they are well blended.
- Serve on top of your salad or as a spread in your favorite sandwiches. This recipe also makes a great dip for raw vegetables.

Dinner Recipes

Now we get to the fun part! These are my most delicious and nutritious recipes. Eating all of these recipes will ensure you are consuming antioxidants, omega-3s, vitamins, minerals, and fiber. This combination of meals contains dark leafy greens, a variety of herbs and spices, and many plant-based options.

Pesto Salmon with Zoodles

Low carb and full of protein, fiber, omega-3 fatty acids, and antioxidants, this Pesto Salmon over Zoodles is a nutrition powerhouse recipe. Some of the nutritious stars are the ALA-rich walnuts and flaxseeds and the antioxidant-rich dark leafy greens, zucchini, and nutritional yeast. This recipe also contains healthy spices like fresh garlic and healthy fats like olive oil. It also happens to be creamy and delicious.

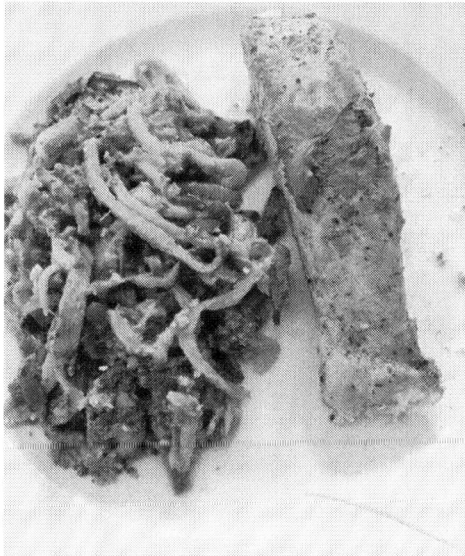

Servings: 4-5

Ingredients for the Pesto Zoodles:

- 2 cups of spinach, washed (You can also use other dark leafy greens like kale, arugula, mustard greens, collard greens, or turnip greens)
- 1/3 cup of Basil
- 1/3 cup of walnuts (You can also use other nuts like almonds, pistachios, cashews, pine)
- 1/4 cup of ground flaxseeds (You can also use other healthy seeds like pumpkin seeds, Chia seed, or hemp seed)
- 1/2 cup of grated parmesan
- 1/4 cup of nutritional yeast
- 2 cloves of fresh garlic
- 1/2 cup of olive oil
- 1 teaspoon of lemon juice
- 1/4 teaspoon of salt
- 1/4 teaspoon of black pepper
- 4 cups pre-packaged zoodles, fresh or frozen (You can also use a spiralizer to make zoodles out of fresh zucchini)

Instructions for the Pesto Zoodles:

1. Combine all the ingredients in a food processor.
2. Blend the ingredients until the consistency is creamy. If the sauce is not "liquid" enough, you can add more extra virgin olive oil.
3. Spray a medium skillet with non-stick cooking spray.
4. Set aside 1/4 cup of pesto sauce for the salmon, then heat the rest of the pesto sauce and the zoodles on medium-high heat for about 4 minutes or until the zoodles are warm. This may take longer if the zoodles are frozen. For frozen zoodles, I like to slightly defrost the zoodles in the microwave before putting them in the skillet. After microwaving, I also drain a little of the water from the zoodles.

Ingredients for Salmon:

- 2 Salmon Fillets
- 1/4 cup of the above pesto
- 1/3 cup sliced cherry tomatoes

Instructions for Salmon:

1. Preheat oven to 400 degrees.
2. Place salmon in a small casserole dish.
3. Spoon the pesto over the salmon.
4. Top the salmon with sliced cherry tomatoes.
5. Bake the salmon uncovered for 20 minutes or until the salmon is done.

Turmeric Chicken Over Yellow Rice

The star of this meal is turmeric. Turmeric has anti-inflammatory properties and promotes immune health. Turmeric also promotes brain health and may even play a role in reducing the risk of Alzheimer's disease. Another highlight of this meal is the fact that the yellow rice is made using whole-grain brown rice. Brown rice is higher in fiber and nutrients than refined white rice, so it's a good idea to replace white rice with brown rice in your favorite recipes. Brown rice has an earthy, gritty texture but still absorbs the flavors just as white rice does.

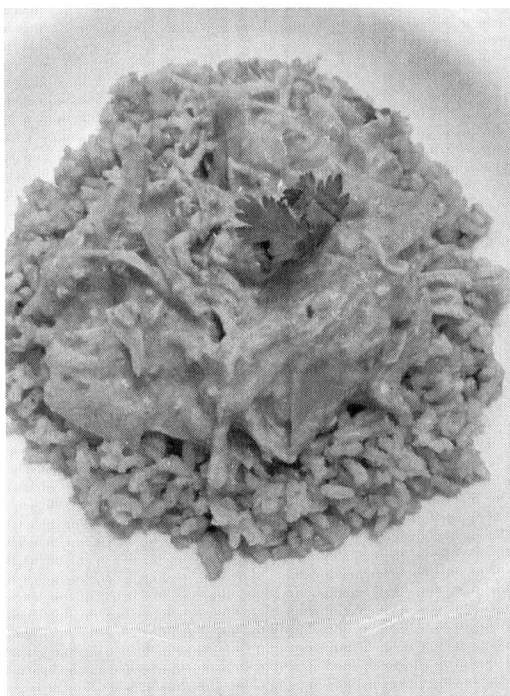

Serves: 8

Materials:

Slow Cooker

Ingredients:

- 2 cups no sugar added tomato sauce
- 1 cup onion, chopped
- 4 cloves garlic, minced
- 1 Tablespoon honey
- 1/2 teaspoon salt
- 1/2 teaspoon black pepper
- 1 Tablespoon Turmeric
- 1 cup scallions, chopped
- 4 oz. cream cheese, softened
- 1 pound boneless, skinless chicken breast, thawed

Instructions for the Turmeric Chicken:

1. Add all ingredients to a large slow cooker.
2. Cook in the slow cooker for 4 to 6 hours.
3. Stir ingredients and break up the chicken when the chicken is tender.

Ingredients for Yellow Rice:

- 2 cups instant brown rice (I like Minute Brown Rice)
- 2 Tablespoons butter
- 3 Tablespoons onion powder
- 1 teaspoon turmeric
- 3 cups vegetable broth
- 1/2 teaspoon salt
- 1/4 teaspoon black pepper
- 3 tablespoons cilantro
- 2 cloves garlic

Instructions for the Turmeric Chicken Over Yellow Rice:

1. Add all the ingredients for the yellow rice to a large pot and bring to a boil.
2. Reduce the heat to low, cover, and simmer for 10 minutes or until the liquid is absorbed.
3. Add 1 cup of yellow rice to a dinner plate. Top with 1 cup of the Turmeric Chicken.

4. Garnish with cilantro, if desired.

Pico De Gallo Cauliflower Rice Bowl

What makes this a Pico De Gallo Rice Bowl a standout recipe? For one, it's low in calories. Two, it's high in nutrients. Three, it's plant-based, and four, it is high in filling fiber. I also recommend adding guacamole to give this recipe extra flavor and nutrition (see recipe above).

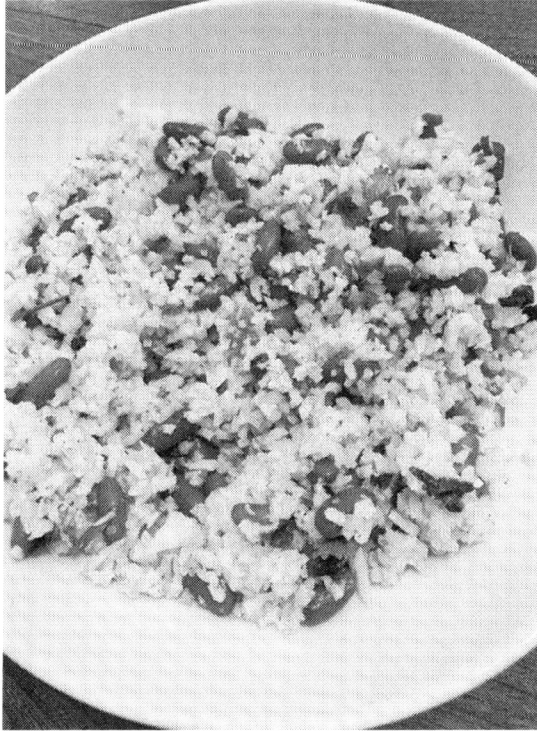

Servings: 6

Ingredients for Pico De Gallo:

- 2 large tomatoes, finely chopped
- 1/4 cup cilantro
- 1 medium jalapeno, finely chopped
- 1/2 white onion, finely chopped
- 1/2 teaspoon salt

- 3 cloves garlic, minced
- 1/4 cup lime juice

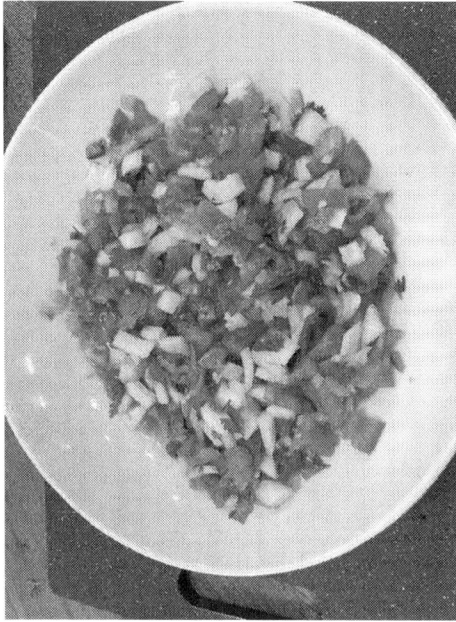

Instructions for Pico De Gallo:

1. Combine all the ingredients in a large bowl.
2. Cover the bowl and set to the side.

*You can also use this recipe alone as a dip. If you decide to make Pico De Gallo for a dip, cover and chill the Pico De Gallo for 30 minutes before serving with your favorite whole-grain tortilla chips.

Ingredients for Cauliflower Rice:

- 4 cups cauliflower rice, frozen
- 1/4 cup lime juice
- 1/4 teaspoon salt
- 3 cloves garlic, minced
- 1/4 cup cilantro
- 1/4 teaspoon cumin
- 1 cup canned kidney beans, drained

- 1 teaspoon Hot Sauce
- 2 teaspoons avocado oil

Instructions for the Pico De Gallo Cauliflower Rice:

1. In a medium skillet, heat oil on medium-high heat for 1 minute.
2. Add all the ingredients to the skillet. Stir ingredients on medium-high heat for 5 to 6 minutes.
3. After you remove the rice for heat, mix in the Pico De Gallo. You can also top this dish with shredded dark leafy greens, cheese, and the guacamole recipe found above.

Ginger Soy Lettuce Wraps

The standout ingredient in this Ginger Soy Lettuce Wrap is ginger. Ginger has anti-inflammatory and antioxidant properties and has been known to soothe an upset stomach. This lettuce wrap is also lower in calories since lettuce is used as the base. In addition, the lean ground chicken provides protein and will help you feel full and satisfied.

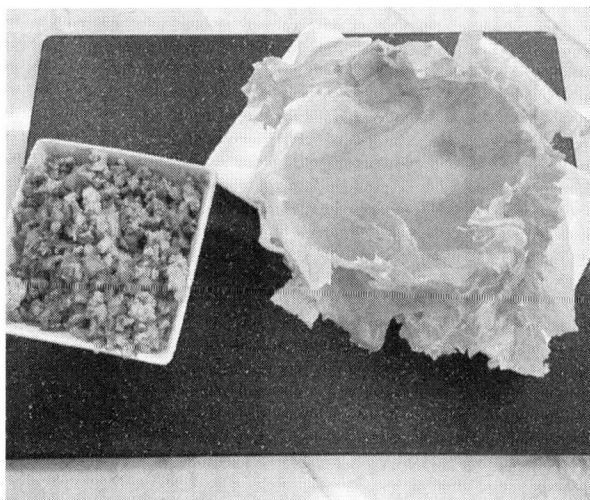

Servings: 3-4

Ingredients:

- 1 pound ground chicken
- 4 cups pre-packaged dry slaw (You can often find a variety of leafy greens in bags of slaw. The bags of slaw are usually located in the produce sections of your grocery store)
- 1/2 teaspoon salt
- 1/4 cup avocado oil
- 1/2 teaspoon black pepper
- 1/2 teaspoon ginger (Make sure the fresh ginger is peeled and grated)
- 3 cloves garlic, minced
- 2 Tablespoons soy sauce, low sodium
- 1/2 teaspoon chili paste
- 1 head of lettuce

Instructions:

- Cook the ground chicken, 1/4 teaspoon salt, 1/4 teaspoon of black pepper, 1/4 teaspoon of ginger, and 1 clove of minced garlic in a medium skillet on medium-high heat for about 9 minutes or until the chicken is no longer pink. While the chicken is cooking, use a spatial to break up and stir the chicken into small bite-size pieces.
- Remove chicken from heat and add one tablespoon of soy sauce and 1/4 teaspoon of chili paste. Stir until the soy sauce, and chili paste is well mixed into the chicken.
- Set the chicken aside.
- Heat avocado oil in a medium skillet on medium-high heat for about 1 minute.
- Add the slaw, 1/4 teaspoon of salt, 1/4 teaspoon of black pepper, 1/4 teaspoon of ginger, 2 cloves of minced garlic. Sauté for about 5 minutes.
- Reduce to low heat and stir in 1 tablespoon of soy sauce and 1/4 teaspoon of chili paste.
- Add the chicken into the slaw. Stir for about 1 minute or until the chicken and slaw is evenly mixed and warm.
- Wash and pat the lettuce dry with a paper towel.

- Carefully pull off each individual leaf. Keep each leaf as whole as possible, but some will probably tear a little, and that is okay.
- To make a lettuce wrap, add about a 1/2 cup of the chicken-slaw mixture into a lettuce leaf, and fold the leaf just like you would a traditional wrap.

Spicy Quinoa with Vegetables

This Spicy Quinoa with Vegetables recipe is so incredibly nutritious:

- Plant-based, check.
- Full of antioxidant-rich vegetables, including a dark leafy green, check.
- Made with a healthy whole grain, check.

You can feel confident that your body is getting many nutrients when you eat this flavorful meal.

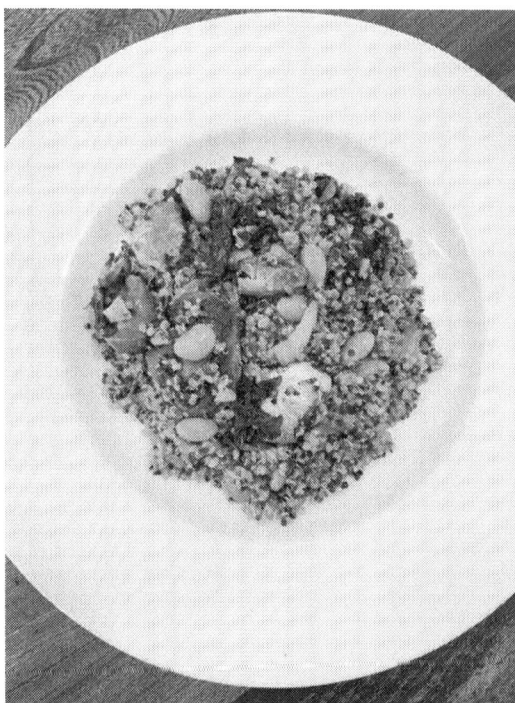

Servings: 4

Ingredients:

- 1 cup quinoa
- 1/2 teaspoon salt
- 1/2 teaspoon pepper

- 4 cloves garlic, minced
- 1/2 cup avocado oil
- 2 cups vegetable broth
- 2 cups Brussel sprout halves
- 2 cups mushrooms, washed and sliced
- 2 cups kale, washed and broken up
- 1 cup onion, chopped
- 1 cup edamame removed from pod before eating
- 1/2 teaspoon Worcestershire sauce
- 1 teaspoon low-sodium soy sauce

Instructions:

1. Pour vegetable broth, 1/4 teaspoon of pepper, and 1/4 teaspoon of salt into a large saucepan and heat to a boil.
2. When the liquid reaches a boil, reduce to low heat and cover. Let the quinoa simmer on low heat for 12 minutes.
3. Remove the quinoa from heat and let it stand covered for about 15 minutes. Set aside.
4. With hot water, thoroughly wash the Brussel sprouts in a colander for about 1 minute.
5. Cut the bottom ends off the Brussel sprouts; then, cut each in half.
6. Heat 1/4 cup of avocado oil in a medium skillet on medium-high heat for about 1 minute.
7. Place the Brussel sprouts face down in the skillet for about 1 minute, then flip each Brussel sprout. Cook the other side on medium-high heat for another minute.
8. Sprinkle 1/4 teaspoon of salt, 1/4 teaspoon of black pepper, and 1 teaspoon of Montreal Steak Seasoning onto the Brussel sprouts and stir the Brussel sprouts over medium heat for about 1 minute. Set the Brussel sprouts aside.
9. Now cook the other vegetables by first heating 1/4 cup of avocado oil in a medium skillet on medium-high heat for about 1 minute.
10. Place the mushrooms, kale, onion, and edamame in the skillet on medium-high heat. Sprinkle with 1/4 teaspoon of salt, 1 teaspoon of Montreal Steak Seasoning, and 3 cloves of fresh garlic, minced. Stir continuously for about 4 minutes.

11. Pour 1 teaspoon of Worcestershire and 1 teaspoon of low salt soy sauce over the vegetables. Stir in thoroughly and remove the vegetables from heat.
12. Combine the quinoa, vegetables, and Brussel sprouts. Remove the edamame from the pods before eating the quinoa bowl.

Breakfast Bowl for Dinner

Think of your classic breakfast bowl with hashbrown potatoes, sausage, and eggs smothered in cheese. This recipe is like that, only with a healthier twist. The palmini noodles take the place of the potatoes, and the ground chicken takes the place of the sausage. This Breakfast Bowl for Dinner also has more vegetables and vitamins, and minerals than the classic version.

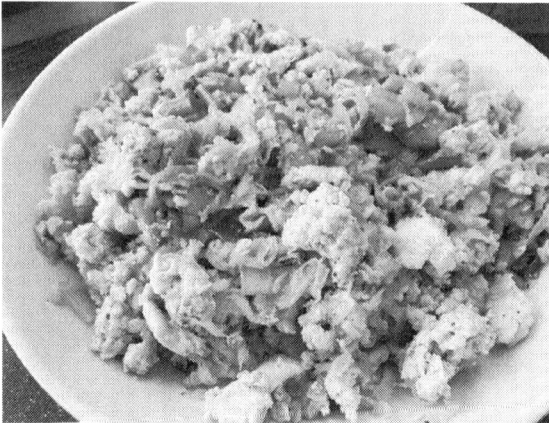

Servings: 4

Ingredients for Turkey Sausage:

- 1 pound lean ground turkey
- 1 teaspoon fennel seeds
- 1 teaspoon Montreal steak seasoning

Ingredients:

- 4 cups palmini noodles
- 1 cup mushrooms, sliced
- 1/2 cup scallions, chopped
- 1/2 cup white onion, chopped
- 1 pound turkey sausage
- 1/2 cup red, orange, and yellow sweet peppers, finely chopped
- 1/2 teaspoon salt
- 1/4 teaspoon black pepper
- 2 Tablespoons hot sauce
- 4 eggs
- 1 cup shredded cheddar cheese
- 1/2 cup avocado oil
- Nonstick cooking spray

Instructions:

1. Cook the ground turkey, fennel seeds, and Montreal seasoning in a medium skillet on medium-high heat for about 9 minutes or until the turkey is no longer pink. While the turkey is cooking, use a spatial to break up and stir the turkey into small bite-size pieces. Remove from heat and drain the excess fat. Set the turkey aside.
2. Whisk the eggs in a small bowl until the yolk and whites are well blended. Stir in 1/4 teaspoon of salt.
3. Heat nonstick cooking spray in a medium skillet on medium-high heat for about 1 minute.
4. Slowly pour the eggs onto the skillet. Continuously stir the eggs until they are light and fluffy. Remove the eggs from the skillet and set aside.
5. In a skillet, heat 1/4 cup of avocado oil for 1 minute.
6. Add the mushrooms, scallions, peppers, 1/4 teaspoon salt, and 1/4 teaspoon of black pepper to the skillet. Sauté the vegetables by frequently stirring them while they cook. When they are done, add 1 tablespoon of hot sauce and remove the vegetables from heat.
7. Heat 1/4 cup of avocado oil in another skillet for 1 minute. (You can wash your original skillet and use it again if you

would like). You just want to make sure the oil used to cook the vegetables is either cleaned out for not overly cooked or close to burning.

8. Place the palmini in the skillet. Stir in 1/4 teaspoon of salt, 1/4 teaspoon black pepper, and 1 Tablespoon of hot sauce. Heat and stir the palmini for about 3 minutes.
9. Combine all the other ingredients (vegetables, cheese, and turkey sausage) with the turnips and serve.

Salmon Cloud Bread Tacos

I have included a few cloud bread recipes because cloud bread is low in calories and has a wonderfully light texture. It's also just fun to make. I really enjoy using cloud bread in recipes because it lets the flavors of the other ingredients shine. The omega-3-rich salmon and guacamole flavors get their time in the spotlight for this cloud bread recipe. For best results, make the cloud bread first, then the salmon, then the guacamole so that the guacamole is nice and fresh. In a pinch, you can also buy store-bought guacamole.

Servings: 4

Materials:

- Parchment paper
- Basting brush

Ingredients for Cloud Bread:

- 1 cup egg whites
- 1 Tablespoon corn starch
- Non-stick cooking spray
- 1 teaspoon olive oil

Instructions for Cloud Bread:

1. Preheat oven to 300 degrees.

2. Beat the egg whites in an electric mixer on high speed until the eggs are light and fluffy.
3. Add in the corn starch and beat in on high speed until the corn starch is well blended.
4. Line a baking sheet with parchment paper; then, spray the paper with non-stick cooking spray.
5. Spread the egg mixture evenly over the parchment paper.
6. Bake for 25 minutes. Then remove the cloud bread from the heat
7. Baste the cloud bread with olive oil and set aside.

Ingredients for the Salmon:

- 4 small salmon fillets
- 3/4 teaspoon salt
- 3/4 teaspoon black pepper
- 3/4 teaspoon Montreal steak seasoning
- 1 Tablespoon lime juice
- 1 Tablespoon lemon juice
- 3 Tablespoons butter

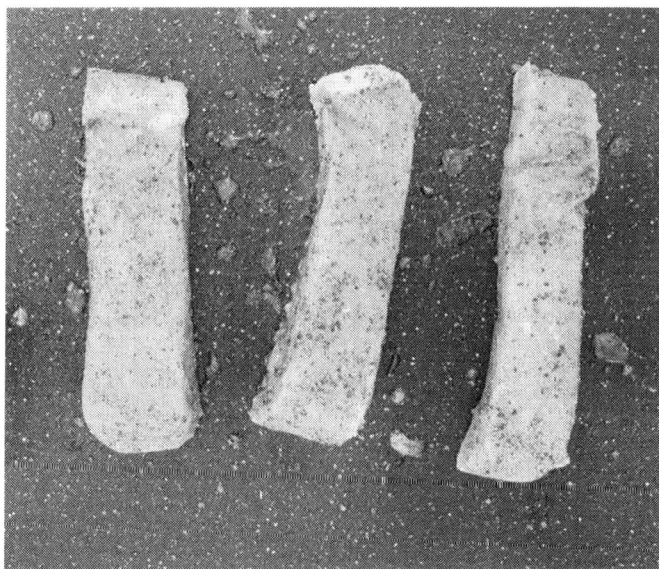

Instructions for the Salmon:

- Combine the lemon juice, lime juice, salt, and pepper in a small bowl.
- Baste each salmon fillet with the lemon-lime juice using a basting brush
- In a medium skillet, melt the butter on medium-high heat.
- Once the butter is melted, place each salmon in the skillet, skin side down.
- Cook for 3 to 4 minutes on medium-high heat; then flip the salmon to the other side.
- Cook the other side on medium-high heat for 3 to 4 minutes or until the salmon is fully cooked. Set aside.

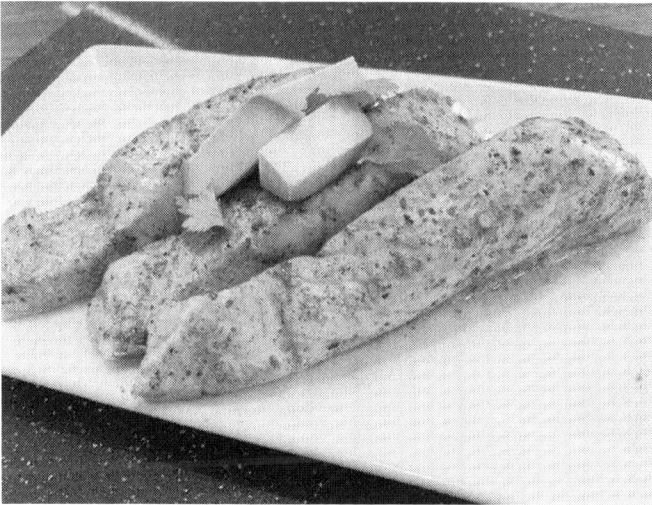

Ingredients for the Guacamole:

- 4 avocados, peeled and pitted
- 2 large tomatoes, finely chopped
- 1/2 cup cilantro
- 1 medium jalapeno, finely chopped
- 1/2 white onion, finely chopped
- 1/4 cup cucumber, finely chopped
- 1/2 teaspoon salt
- 4 cloves garlic, minced
- 1/2 cup lime juice

Instructions for the Guacamole:

1. Combine all the ingredients in a large bowl. Mash and stir the ingredients together until the avocado is smashed to your liking. (Some like chunky guacamole, and others like creamy guacamole. I like mine a little chunky). Set aside.

Instructions for Building the Salmon Cloud Bread Tacos:

1. Cut the cloud bread into smaller rectangles. It should make about 3 to 4 tacos, depending on how big you want your tacos.
2. Remove thc skin from the salmon and cut up the salmon into bite-size pieces.
3. Add the salmon to the cloud bread and top with the guacamole.
4. Fold the cloud bread into a "taco" around the salmon.

Konjac Noodles with Vegetables

Konjac pasta comes from the konjac yam and contains mostly water and fiber. In fact, one serving of konjac pasta is only about ten calories. So, this Konjac Noodles with Vegetables recipe is low in calories and high in fiber and other nutrients. It's also another entirely plant-based recipe, yet still high in protein thanks to the nutritional yeast.

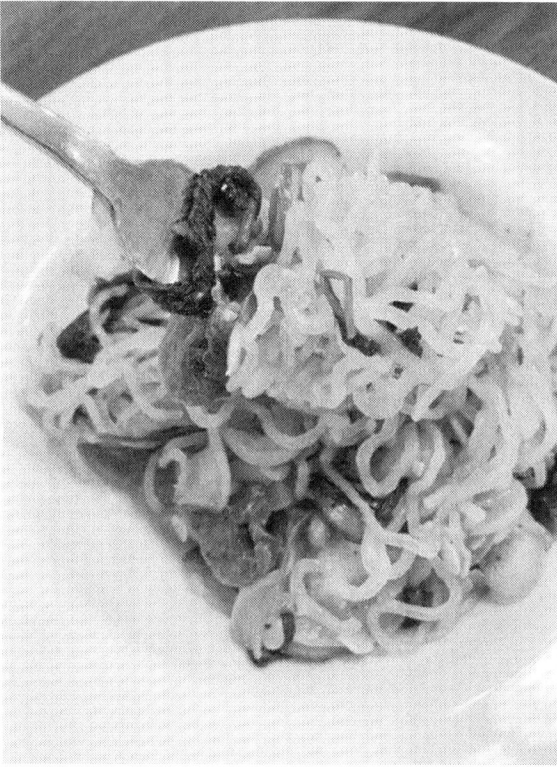

Servings: 4

Ingredients:

- 2 cups mushrooms, sliced
- 4 cup spinach leaves
- 2 cups zucchini, sliced
- 2 cups squash, sliced
- 2 cups onion, chopped
- 4 cloves garlic, minced
- 1/2 Tablespoon Worcestershire
- 1 Tablespoon soy sauce, low sodium
- 1 Tablespoon Montreal steak seasoning
- 1 cup vegetable broth
- 1 Tablespoon nutritional yeast
- 1/4 cup avocado oil
- 1/4 teaspoon salt
- 1/4 teaspoon black pepper

- 400 g or 14 oz. konjac pasta

Instructions:

1. Prepare konjac noodles per package directions and set them aside.
2. In a large skillet, heat avocado oil for one minute.
3. Add in the squash, zucchini, onions, mushrooms, and fresh garlic. Sprinkle with salt, pepper, and Montreal steak seasoning.
4. Stir frequently on medium-high heat for about 5 minutes.
5. Remove the vegetables from heat; then stir in the soy sauce and Worcestershire sauce.
6. Reduce heat to low and stir in konjac pasta, vegetable broth, and nutritional yeast.
7. Stir on low heat for about 3 minutes or until the konjac pasta is warm.

Supreme Cloud Bread Pizza

The low-calorie cloud bread makes another appearance on this meal plan, but this time in the form of pizza instead of tacos. Pizza toppings provide you with the opportunity to add a multitude of nutritious vegetables. We also topped this pizza with turkey "sausage" to give this pizza a little protein kick.

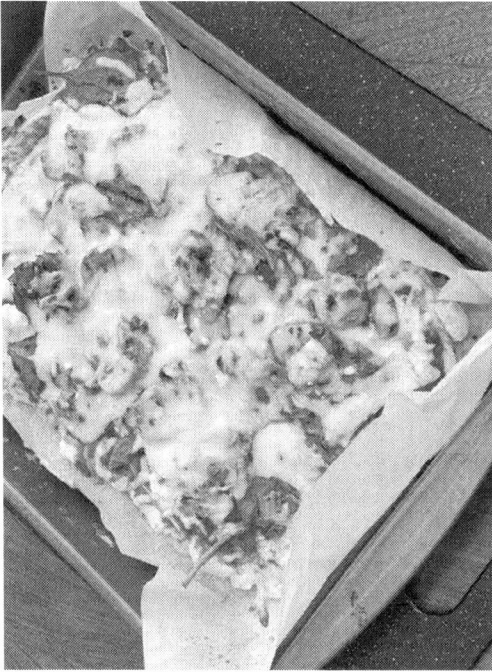

Servings: 1

Materials:

- Parchment paper
- Basting brush

Ingredients for Cloud Bread:

- 1 cup egg whites
- 1 Tablespoon corn starch
- Non-stick cooking spray
- 1 teaspoon extra virgin olive oil

Instructions for Cloud Bread:

- Preheat oven to 300 degrees.
- Beat the egg whites in an electric mixer on high speed until the eggs are light and fluffy.

- Add in the corn starch and beat in on high speed until the corn starch is well blended.
- Line a baking sheet with parchment paper; then, spray the paper with non-stick cooking spray.
- Spread the egg mixture evenly over the parchment paper.
- Bake for 25 minutes. Then remove the cloud bread from heat.
- Baste the cloud bread with olive oil and set aside.

Ingredients for Cloud Bread Supreme Pizza:

- Cloud bread (from the above recipe)
- 2 Tablespoons extra virgin olive oil
- 2 Tablespoons avocado oil
- 1/2 cup no sugar added tomato sauce
- 1 cup fresh spinach leaves
- 1/2 cup mushrooms, sliced
- 1/3 cup green peppers
- 1/3 cup canned black olives, chopped
- 2 cloves garlic, minced
- 1/4 cup onions, chopped
- 1 Tablespoon oregano
- 1 teaspoon crushed red pepper flakes
- 1 Tablespoon parsley
- 1 cup mozzarella cheese, shredded
- 1/2 pound of ground turkey
- 1/2 teaspoon fennel seeds
- 1 teaspoon Montreal steak seasoning

Instructions for Cloud Bread Supreme Pizza:

- Preheat the oven to 375 degrees.
- Cook the ground turkey, fennel seeds, and Montreal seasoning in a medium skillet on medium-high heat for about 9 minutes or until the turkey is no longer pink. While the turkey is cooking, use a spatial to break up and stir the turkey into small bite-size pieces. Remove from heat and drain the excess fat. Set the turkey aside.
- Heat 2 Tablespoons of avocado oil in a medium skillet on high heat for about 1 minute.

- Reduce heat to medium-high, and add mushrooms, peppers, garlic, onions, oregano, parsley, and crushed red pepper flakes to the skillet. Stir ingredients on medium-high heat for about 2 minutes. Remove ingredients from the heat and set aside.
- Using a basting brush, spread 2 Tablespoons of extra virgin olive oil on the top of the cloud bread.
- Using the same basting brush, evenly spread the tomato sauce on the top of the cloud bread.
- Add the spinach leaves to the bread.
- Evenly sprinkle the turkey sausage all over the pizza.
- Evenly sprinkle the olives and the mushroom, onion, spice mixture on top of the cloud bread.
- Finally, add a layer of mozzarella cheese.
- Bake in the oven for 10 minutes.

Chickpeas and Turmeric Over Yellow Rice

This Chickpea Tikka Masala Over Yellow Rice is a high protein, plant-based winner. My favorite ingredient in this recipe is turmeric. I wanted to make sure I included the turmeric spice in some of these meals because turmeric is just so good for us. I also love that the yellow rice is made with fiber-rich whole-grain brown rice instead of refined white rice. Note that the tomato sauce in the ingredients list says no sugar added. Try to look for no sugar added sauces and condiments whenever you go grocery shopping.

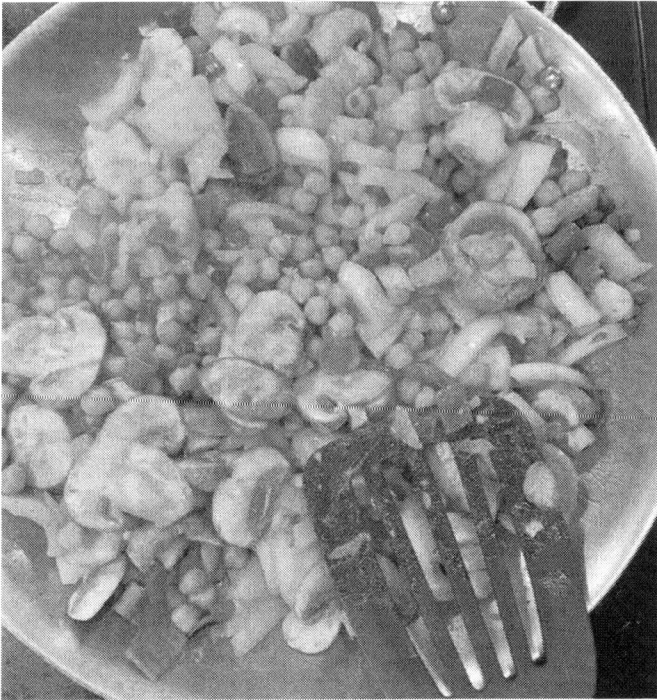

Ingredients for Chickpeas and Turmeric:

- 1 1/2 cups no sugar added tomato sauce
- 1 cup onion, chopped
- 4 cloves garlic, minced
- 1 Tablespoon honey
- 1/2 teaspoon salt
- 1/2 teaspoon black pepper
- 1 Tablespoon turmeric
- 1 cup scallions, chopped
- 4 oz. light cream cheese, softened (You can also use vegan cream cheese to make this a completely vegan recipe)
- 1 cup mushrooms, sliced
- 1/4 cup capers
- 1/4 cup avocado oil
- 15.5 oz canned chickpeas

Instructions for Chickpeas and Turmeric:

1. Heat the avocado oil on medium-high heat for 1 minute.
2. Add chickpeas, mushrooms, onions, garlic, scallions, turmeric, capers, salt, and pepper to the saucepan. Stir frequently for about 4 minutes.
3. Add in the no sugar added tomato sauce, honey, and cream cheese. Stir for about 1 minute or until the cream cheese is well blended into the sauce.
4. Serve on top of yellow rice. The yellow rice recipe is below.

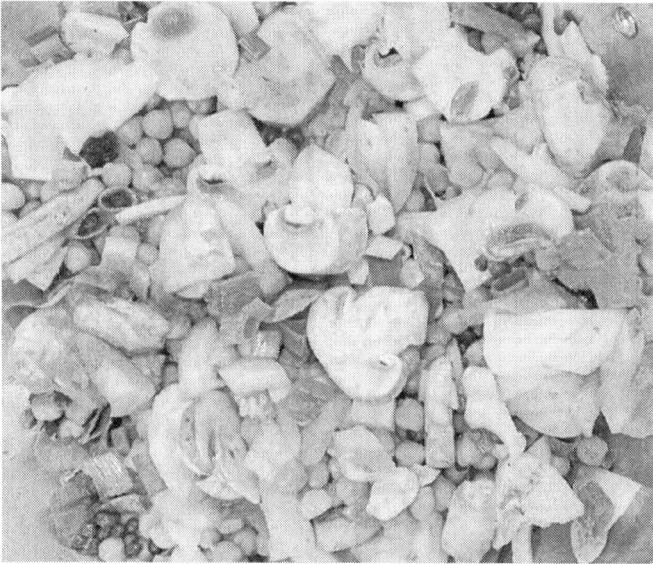

Ingredients for Yellow Rice:

- 2 cups instant brown rice (I like Minute Brown Rice)
- 2 Tablespoons butter
- 3 Tablespoons onion powder
- 1 teaspoon turmeric
- 3 cups vegetable broth
- 1/2 teaspoon salt
- 1/4 teaspoon black pepper
- 3 tablespoons cilantro
- 2 cloves garlic

Instructions for Chickpea Turmeric Over Yellow Rice:

1. Add all the ingredients for the yellow rice to a large pot and bring to a boil.
2. Reduce the heat to low, cover, and simmer for 10 minutes or until the liquid is absorbed.
3. Add 1 cup of yellow rice to a dinner plate. Top with 1 cup of the Chickpea Turmeric.
4. Garnish with cilantro, if desired.

Taco Pasta

Hearty and comforting, with a cheesy southwest flair, this taco pasta is a hit with young and old. The Taco Pasta is healthier than traditional pasta, thanks to the palmini. Palmini is a low-calorie alternative to white pasta. You can also use whole-grain pasta as another healthier alternative. Just remember to cook the pasta per package directions before adding the pasta to your casserole dish.

Serves 6

Materials:

- 9" x13" pans (aluminum, or disposable)
- Plastic wrap
- Aluminum foil

Ingredients:

- 1 pound ground turkey
- 1 packet taco seasoning
- 4 ounces cream cheese, light
- 4 cups palmini pasta
- 8 oz jar of salsa
- 8 oz jar of taco sauce (2 cups)
- 1 cup light sharp cheddar cheese, grated
- 1 cup mozzarella cheese, grated

Instructions:

- Preheat the oven to 350 degrees.
- Cook the ground turkey, fennel seeds, and Montreal seasoning in a medium skillet on medium-high heat for about 9 minutes or until the turkey is no longer pink. While the turkey is cooking, use a spatial to break up and stir the turkey into small bite-size pieces. Remove from heat and drain the excess fat. Set the turkey aside.

- Add taco seasoning and cream cheese to the pan.
- Stir until cream cheese is melted.
- Prepare the palmini pasta per directions on the package.
- Add meat mixture, salsa, cheddar, mozzarella, taco sauce, and pasta to the 9" X 13" pan and stir the ingredients until they are well blended.
- Cover the casserole dish with foil.
- Bake for 1 hour. Remove foil and bake an additional 10-15 minutes.

Chickpea Lettuce Wrap

Remember, people in the blue zones follow 90-100% plant-based diets, so we want our meal plan to be heavily plant-based too. This Chickpea Lettuce Wrap is another one of those delicious plant-based meals that provide plenty of protein. It also happens to be super easy to make. In fact, you don't even have to cook anything!

Servings: 4

Ingredients:

- 1 Tablespoon plain Greek yogurt
- 1 Tablespoon lemon juice
- 1/2 teaspoon sea salt
- 1/2 teaspoon black pepper
- 1 Tablespoon cilantro
- 3 cloves garlic, minced
- 1 teaspoon cayenne pepper
- 1 cup celery, thinly sliced
- 1/2 cup red onions, chopped
- 1/2 cup cherry tomato halves
- 1 cup walnuts, chopped
- 2 Tablespoons extra virgin olive oil
- 1 cup canned chickpeas, drained
- 4 cups of dark leafy greens (ex: kale or spinach), finely shredded
- Head of lettuce

Instructions:

- Combine all ingredients except for the lettuce. Refrigerate until you are ready to serve.
- Wash and pat the lettuce dry with a paper towel.
- Carefully pull off each individual leaf. Keep each leaf as whole as possible, but some will probably tear a little, which is okay.

- To make a lettuce wrap, add about a 1/2 cup of the chickpea salad into a lettuce leaf, and fold the leaf just like you would a traditional wrap.

Vegetable Cloud Bread Pizza

Mushrooms always work well in plant-based recipes like this Vegetable Cloud Bread Pizza because they give the recipe a "meaty" flavor. However, this recipe is also low in calories and high in vitamins, minerals, and antioxidants, thanks to all the vegetables, including those powerhouse dark leafy greens.

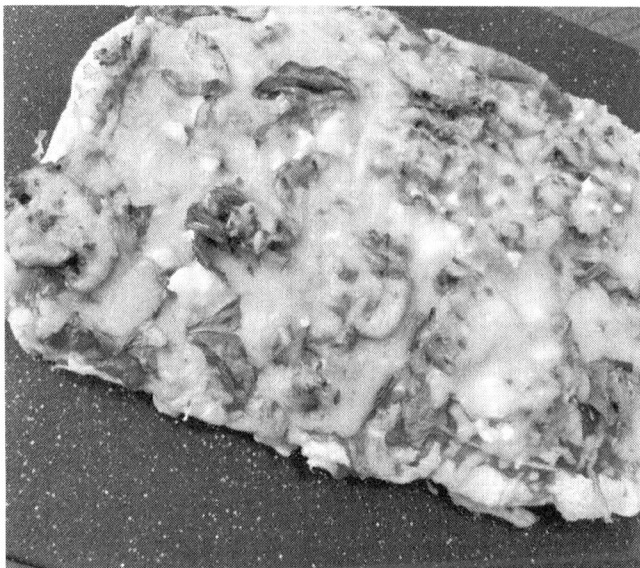

Servings: 1

Materials:

- Parchment paper
- Basting brush

Ingredients for Cloud Bread:

- 1 cup egg whites
- 1 Tablespoon corn starch
- Non-stick cooking spray

Instructions for Cloud Bread:

1. Preheat oven to 300 degrees.
2. Beat Egg whites in an electric mixer on high speed until the eggs are light and fluffy.
3. Add in the corn starch and beat in on high speed until the corn starch is well blended.
4. Line a baking sheet with parchment paper; then, spray the paper with non-stick cooking spray.
5. Spread the egg mixture evenly over the parchment paper.
6. Bake for 25 minutes. Then remove the cloud bread from heat and set aside.

Ingredients for Cloud Bread Vegetable Pizza:

- Cloud bread (from the above recipe)
- 2 Tablespoons extra virgin olive oil
- 2 Tablespoons avocado oil
- 1 cup fresh spinach leaves
- 1/2 cup mushrooms, sliced
- 1/2 cup canned artichoke hearts
- 2 cloves garlic, minced
- 1/4 cup onions, chopped
- 1/2 cup no sugar added tomato sauce
- 1 Tablespoon oregano
- 1 teaspoon crushed red pepper flakes
- 1 Tablespoon parsley
- 1 cup mozzarella cheese, shredded
- 1/3 cup feta cheese crumbles

Instructions for Cloud Bread Vegetable Pizza:

- Preheat the oven to 375 degrees.
- Heat 2 Tablespoons of avocado oil in a medium skillet on high heat for about 1 minute.
- Reduce heat to medium-high, and add mushrooms, garlic, onions, oregano, parsley, and crushed red pepper flakes to the skillet. Stir ingredients on medium-high heat for about 2 minutes. Remove ingredients from the heat and set aside.
- Using a basting brush, spread 2 Tablespoons of extra virgin olive oil on the top of the cloud bread.

- Using the same basting brush, evenly spread the tomato sauce on the top of the cloud bread.
- Add the spinach leaves to the bread.
- Evenly sprinkle the feta cheese and the mushroom, onion, spice mixture on top of the cloud bread.
- Finally, add a layer of mozzarella cheese.
- Bake in the oven for 10 minutes.

Chicken Lo Mein

It's simple, low in calories, high in protein, and delicious! I love all the textures and flavors in this Chicken Lo Mein. The high-fiber, low-calorie konjac noodles make this recipe unique and give it that silky glass noodles texture. Remember, when buying sauces, look for the no added sugar version. For this recipe, you will need no sugar added ketchup.

Servings: 4

Materials:

- Skillet
- Meat Tenderizer

Ingredients:

- 1/4 cup avocado oil
- 1 pound chicken, skinless, boneless, thawed, and cut into bite-size pieces
- 1 cup scallions, diced
- 3 cloves garlic, minced
- 4 Tablespoons honey
- 1/2 cup soy sauce, low sodium
- 1/3 cup no sugar added ketchup
- 1/4 teaspoon salt
- 1/4 teaspoon pepper
- 4 cups konjac pasta

Instructions:

- Tenderized chicken by beating it with tenderizer for one minute on both sides.
- Sprinkle the chicken with salt and pepper or use a basting brush to brush salt and pepper onto the chicken.
- Heat avocado oil in a medium skillet on medium-high heat for about one minute.

- Place chicken evenly on the skillet. Let the chicken cook on one side for about 1 minute; then, flip each piece of chicken. Let the chicken cook for one minute on the other side.
- Reduce the heat to low heat and add the soy, scallions, garlic, honey, soy sauce, and ketchup. Stir until the ingredients are well blended.
- Prepare the konjac pasta per package directions, then add the pasta to the skillet mixture. Stir and heat for 1 minute or until the konjac pasta is warm.

Pesto Pasta

I included several recipes with this powerhouse pesto because it is packed with so many healthy ingredients- nuts, seeds, nutritional yeast, and dark leafy greens. This pasta has it all! This time the pasta is served over zoodle pasta and topped with tomatoes and mushrooms.

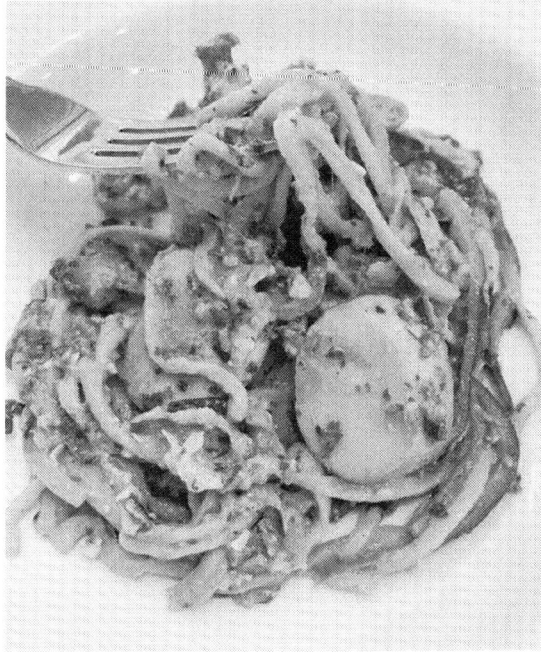

Servings: 4-5

Ingredients for the Pesto Sauce:

- 2 cups spinach, washed (You can also use other dark leafy greens like kale, arugula, mustard greens, collard greens, or turnip greens)
- 1/3 cup basil
- 1/3 cup walnuts (You can also use other nuts like almonds, pistachios, cashews, pine)
- 1/4 cup ground flaxseeds (You can also use other healthy seeds like pumpkin seeds, Chia seed, or hemp seed)

- 1/2 cup grated parmesan
- 1/4 cup nutritional yeast
- 2 cloves fresh garlic
- 1/2 cup olive oil
- 1 teaspoon lemon juice
- 1/4 teaspoon salt
- 1/4 teaspoon black pepper
- 4 cups pre-packaged zoodles, fresh or frozen (You can also use a spiralizer to make zoodles out of fresh zucchini)

Instructions for the Pesto:

- Combine all the ingredients in a food processor.
- Blend the ingredients until the consistency is creamy. If the sauce is not "liquid" enough, you can add more extra virgin olive oil. Set the pesto aside.

Ingredients for the Pesto Pasta:

- 1 cup pesto sauce
- 1 cup sliced cherry tomatoes
- 2 cups sliced mushrooms, washed
- 2 1/2 cups whole-grain pasta, cooked (You can also use other healthy pasta like veggie pasta, chickpea pasta, buckwheat pasta, zoodles, etc.)

Instructions:

1. Combine pesto sauce, mushrooms, cherry tomatoes, and cooked pasta in a pan and heat on medium-high heat for 5 minutes, or until the pesto and pasta are warm.
2. Cover the pan and remove the pan from the heat.
3. Let the pesto pasta sit while covered for 5 minutes.

Mushroom Soup

I love this comforting, creamy, and warm mushroom soup. To add a crunch, you can top this soup with your favorite whole-grain cracker crumbles. You can also add a cup of nutritional yeast to sneak in a complete protein.

Servings: 6

Ingredients:

- 4 cups vegetable broth
- 6 cups mushrooms, sliced
- 2 cups water
- 1 Tablespoon butter
- 1 Tablespoon extra-virgin olive oil
- 1 cup scallions, chopped (about 4 scallions)
- 2 stalks celery, chopped
- 4 cloves garlic, minced
- 1/2 teaspoon salt
- 1/2 teaspoon black pepper
- 2 Tablespoons cornstarch
- 1/2 cup light sour cream

Instructions:

- Melt the butter in a medium skillet on medium-high heat. Add the mushrooms, scallions, celery, salt, pepper, and garlic to the skillet. Cook and stir for about 5 minutes. Slowly stir in the cornstarch and 1 cup of broth for about 2 minutes or until the cornstarch is evenly mixed into the vegetables.
- Combine all the ingredients in a large pot and bring to a boil.
- Reduce heat to low heat and simmer for about 20 minutes. Occasionally stir the soup.

Turkey Chili

A meal plan is not complete without a few comforting soups, like this protein-packed Turkey Chili. The ingredients that make this recipe healthier than traditional chili are the lean turkey and the no sugar added tomato sauce. In addition, kidney beans, mushrooms, onions, and garlic provide lots of vitamins, minerals, and antioxidants.

Servings: 6

Ingredients:

- 1 pound lean ground turkey
- 1 small yellow onion, peeled and chopped (1 cup)
- 1 1/2 cup mushrooms, sliced
- 1 cup cans kidney beans, drained and rinsed
- 24 oz no sugar added tomato sauce
- 4 large cloves of garlic, minced
- 1 Tablespoon chili powder

Instructions:

- Cook the ground turkey on medium-high heat for about 9 minutes or until the turkey is no longer pink. While the turkey is cooking, use a spatial to break up and stir the turkey into small bite-size pieces. Remove from heat and drain the excess fat. Set the turkey aside.
- In a large pot, combine the turkey with all the other remaining ingredients and bring to a boil.
- Reduce heat, cover, and simmer for about 10 minutes. Occasionally lift the lid and stir the soup.

Pesto Pizza Tortilla

Previous pizza recipes in this meal plan used cloud bread as the base, but this one uses whole-wheat tortillas as the base. Of course, you can always go back to using the cloud bread as a base as well, if you prefer.

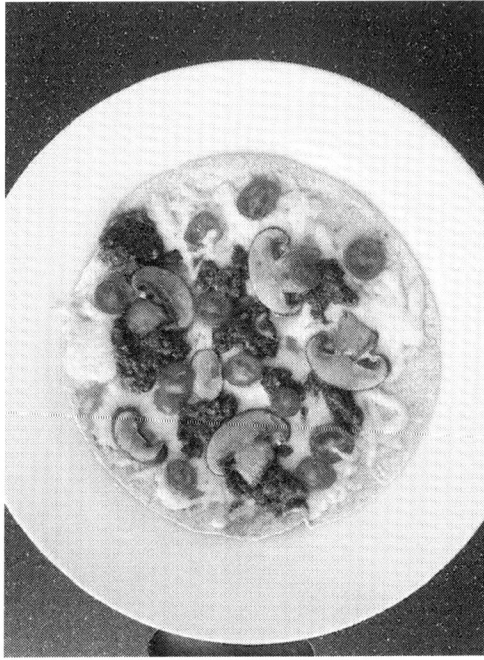

Servings: 4

Ingredients for the Pesto Sauce:

- 2 cups spinach, washed (You can also use other dark leafy greens like kale, arugula, mustard greens, collard greens, or turnip greens)
- 1/3 cup basil
- 1/3 cup walnuts (You can also use other nuts like almonds, pistachios, cashews, pine)
- 1/4 cup ground flaxseeds (You can also use other healthy seeds like pumpkin seeds, Chia seed, or hemp seed)
- 1/2 cup grated parmesan
- 1/4 cup nutritional yeast
- 2 cloves fresh garlic
- 1/2 cup olive oil
- 1 teaspoon lemon juice
- 1/4 teaspoon salt
- 1/4 teaspoon black pepper
- 4 cups pre-packaged zoodles, fresh or frozen (You can also use a spiralizer to make zoodles out of fresh zucchini)

Instructions for the Pesto:

- Combine all the ingredients in a food processor.
- Blend the ingredients until the consistency is creamy. If the sauce is not "liquid" enough, you can add more extra virgin olive oil. Set the pesto aside.

Ingredients for the Pesto Pizza Tortilla:

- Pesto sauce (Use about 1/3 cup for each tortilla, but the amount can vary based on your sauce to pizza ratio preferences)
- 3 sliced cherry tomatoes
- 1 sliced baby Bella mushrooms, washed
- 1/2 teaspoon extra virgin olive oil
- 1/2 cup of mozzarella cheese, shredded
- 4 whole-grain soft tortilla

Instructions:

1. Preheat the oven to 250 degrees.
2. Place the tortilla wrap flat on a baking sheet.
3. Brush the tortilla wraps with the extra virgin olive oil using a basting brush.
4. Evenly sprinkle the mozzarella cheese on top of the tortilla.
5. Top the tortilla with scoops for pesto sauce. Try to space the pesto scoops evenly.
6. Evenly top the tortilla with cherry tomatoes and mushrooms.
7. Bake uncovered in the oven for 8 minutes.

Fish Tacos

I love using pre-packaged slaw in recipes! They are so easy and convenient, and you can often find slaw packs with a variety of healthy vegetables like kale, carrots, cabbage, and spinach. You enhance the slaw packs by adding a little red onion, lime juice, and salt to this recipe.

Servings: 6

Ingredients for Slaw:

- 1 package pre-chopped, dry slaw mix
- 1 Tablespoon lime juice
- 1/4 teaspoon salt
- 1/2 cup red onion, diced

Instructions for Slaw:

In a large bowl, combine all the slaw ingredients, cover, and chill in the refrigerator until the rest of the recipe steps are completed.

Ingredients for Fish Tacos:

- 4 tilapia fillets
- 1/4 teaspoon ground cayenne pepper
- 1/2 teaspoon cumin
- 3 cloves garlic, minced
- 1/2 teaspoon salt
- 1/2 teaspoon black pepper
- Slaw from the recipe above
- 12 whole-grain tortillas
- 1 cup fresh cilantro leaves

Instructions for Fish Tacos:

- In a large bowl, mix the cayenne pepper, cumin, garlic, salt, and black pepper.

- With a basting brush, brush the seasoning mixture on the top and bottom of each fish fillet.
- Spray a medium skillet with non-stick cooking spray and heat on medium-high heat for 1 minute.
- Evenly place the fish fillets in the skillet and cook one side down for about 4 minutes.
- Flip the fillet and cook the other side for another 4 minutes.
- Reduce the heat to low. Then using a fork, break apart the fillets into bite-size pieces. You will also be able to see if the fish is completely done on the inside.
- Place each tortilla on the skillet (it should still be warm) for about 1 minute.
- Remove the fish from heat. Fill each tortilla with the fish and slaw.
- Garnish with lime juice and cilantro.

Palmini Lasagna

You can now get cans or pouches of palmini shaped like lasagna sheets. For this recipe, combine these low-calorie palmini sheets with lean ground turkey and add some frozen spinach to get a healthier version of a family classic.

Servings: 6

Materials:

- 9" x13" pans (glass, aluminum, or disposable)
- Aluminum foil

Ingredients:

- 1 pound ground turkey- cooked
- 2 large eggs
- 15 oz ricotta cheese
- 1 cup shredded parmesan cheese
- 8 oz mozzarella cheese, freshly shredded and divided in half
- 2 teaspoons salt

- 1 teaspoon pepper
- 24 oz jar no sugar added pasta sauce
- 2 cups frozen spinach, chopped (about 3 cups)
- 8 oz. palmini lasagna sheets

Instructions:

- Preheat the oven to 375 degrees.
- Prepare the palmini lasagna per package directions.
- Cook the ground turkey in a medium skillet on medium-high heat for about 9 minutes or until the turkey is no longer pink. While the turkey is cooking, use a spatial to break up and stir the turkey into small bite-size pieces. Remove from heat and drain the excess fat. Set the turkey aside.
- In a large bowl, create cheese filling by combining eggs, ricotta, parmesan, half of the mozzarella cheese, parsley, salt, and pepper.
- Spread a thin layer of pasta sauce at the bottom of the casserole dish. For the next layer, add palmini lasagna noodles. Next, add 1/2 the cheese filling. Then spread 1 cup the frozen spinach. For the next layer, sprinkle with cooked ground turkey. Now spread a layer of pasta sauce again and repeat the other layers one more time.
- Add mozzarella cheese on top.
- Cover the dish with foil and bake for about 16 minutes or until the center is warm. Remove foil and bake for additional 5 minutes or until cheese on top is melted.

Pesto Grilled Cheese on Wheat

Grilled cheese makes me think of my childhood, but now I crave a more grown-up version. This gooey melted cheese, spinach, and mushroom sandwich is perfect for these grown-up taste buds.

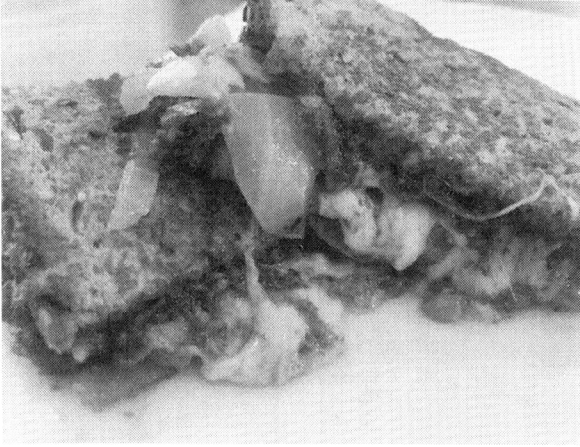

Servings: 4

Ingredients for the Pesto Sauce:

- 2 cups spinach, washed (You can also use other dark leafy greens like kale, arugula, mustard greens, collard greens, or turnip greens)
- 1/3 cup basil
- 1/3 cup walnuts (You can also use other nuts like almonds, pistachios, cashews, pine)
- 1/4 cup ground flaxseeds (You can also use other healthy seeds like pumpkin seeds, Chia seed, or hemp seed)
- 1/2 cup grated parmesan
- 1/4 cup nutritional yeast
- 2 cloves fresh garlic
- 1/2 cup olive oil
- 1 teaspoon lemon juice
- 1/4 teaspoon salt
- 1/4 teaspoon black pepper
- 4 cups pre-packaged zoodles, fresh or frozen (You can also use a spiralizer to make zoodles out of fresh zucchini)

Instructions for the Pesto:

- Combine all the ingredients in a food processor.

- Blend the ingredients until the consistency is creamy. If the sauce is not "liquid" enough, you can add more extra virgin olive oil. Set the pesto aside.

Ingredients:

- 1/2 cup chopped onion
- 1 mushroom, sliced
- 2 cherry tomatoes, sliced
- 1/3 cup pesto sauce
- 1/3 cup mozzarella cheese, shredded
- 8 slices whole wheat bread
- Non-stick cooking spray

Instructions:

1. Bring a pan to medium-high heat on the stovetop. Let the pan heat for about 1 minute.
2. Spray the pan with cooking oil. Let the cooking oil heat for about 1 minute.
3. Add the onion, cherry tomatoes, and mushrooms to the pan, and sauté for about 3 minutes. Remove the pan from the heat. Set the pan aside to use later.
4. On a plate, add the pesto, mozzarella cheese, and sautéed vegetables to one slice of bread.
5. Top with another slice of bread.
6. Spray the pan again with olive oil. Preheat the pan again on medium-high heat for 2 minutes.
7. Place the sandwich on the pan and cover for 2 minutes.
8. Uncover, then flip the sandwich.
9. Press the sandwich with a spatula.
10. Cover the pan with a lid again for 2 more minutes.
11. Repeat this to make the other 3 sandwiches.

*Note cook times will vary.

Taco Chili

Chili with a twist, this Taco Chili provides ample protein, vitamins, and minerals. We use lean turkey, peppers, onions, black beans, corn, and no sugar added tomato sauce for this chili recipe. The seasoning is simple, just one tablespoon of taco seasoning adds plenty of flavors.

Servings: 6

Ingredients:

- 1 pound ground turkey
- 1 small yellow onion, peeled and chopped (1 cup)
- 1 medium-sized green bell pepper, chopped
- 1 cup frozen corn
- 8 oz. can black beans
- 24 oz can no sugar added pasta sauce
- 1 Tablespoon taco seasoning

Instructions:

- Cook the ground turkey in a medium skillet on medium-high heat for about 9 minutes or until the turkey is no longer pink. While the turkey is cooking, use a spatial to break up and stir the turkey into small bite-size pieces. Remove from heat and drain the excess fat. Set the turkey aside.
- Combine all the ingredients in a large pot and bring to a boil.
- Reduce heat to low, cover, and simmer for 20 minutes, stirring occasionally.

Comfort Baked Spaghetti

There are several reasons to love this comforting casserole dish. One, whole grains provide lots of protein, B vitamins, and minerals. Two, the turkey is going to be a leaner alternative to ground beef.

Three, when you use no sugar added tomato sauce, you get less sugar than spaghetti made with many other brands of spaghetti sauce.

Servings: 5

Ingredients:

- 16 oz. package whole-grain spaghetti
- 1-pound lean ground turkey
- 1 onion, chopped
- 32 oz. no sugar added tomato sauce
- 1/2 teaspoon salt
- 1/2 teaspoon black pepper
- 2 eggs
- 3 Tablespoons butter
- 4 cups mozzarella cheese, shredded
- Non-stick cooking spray

Instructions:

- Preheat oven to 350 degrees.
- Cook the ground turkey and onions in a medium skillet on medium-high heat for about 9 minutes or until the turkey is no longer pink. While the turkey is cooking, use a spatial to break up and stir the turkey into small bite-size pieces. Remove from heat and drain the excess fat. Set the turkey aside.
- Cook pasta noodles per package directions.
- Whisk eggs and butter in a large bowl and add in pasta. Toss until the pasta is well coated.
- Mix in spaghetti and the rest of the ingredients with the egg mixture and toss to coat.
- Lightly spray a 9 X 13-inch baking dish with non-stick cooking spray.
- Spread the pasta, meat, egg mixture in the casserole dish. Sprinkle with the mozzarella cheese.
- Cover with foil and bake in the oven for 40 minutes or until the cheese is melted.

Italian Meatball Cloud Bread Sandwich

This is such a fun one and popular with the whole family. The meatballs are made with whole-grain oats, spinach, and lean turkey, making the meatballs extra nutritious. Eating the meatballs on top of cloud bread is just plain fun, not to mention low in calories and high in protein.

Servings: 4 to 6

Materials:

- Parchment paper
- Basting brush

Ingredients for the Meatballs:

- 1 pound lean ground turkey
- 2 large eggs
- 1/2 package onion soup mix
- 4 oz. frozen spinach
- 1/2 cup uncooked old-fashioned oats
- 1 teaspoon Montreal steak seasoning
- 1 teaspoon Worcestershire sauce
- 2 teaspoons salt
- 1/2 teaspoon pepper
- Cooking spray

Instructions for the Meatballs:

- Preheat oven to 400 degrees.
- In a medium-mixing bowl, combine all the ingredients except tomato sauce. Line a baking pan with parchment paper.

- Mold your meat into balls using either your hands or a meat baller.
- Bake at 400 degrees for 30-40 minutes or until internal meatball temperature registers 160 degrees.

Ingredients for Cloud Bread:

- 1 cup egg whites
- 1 Tablespoon corn starch
- Non-stick cooking spray

Instructions for Cloud Bread:

- Preheat oven to 300 degrees.
- Beat egg whites in an electric mixer on high speed until the eggs are light and fluffy.
- Add in the corn starch and beat in on high speed until the corn starch is well blended.
- Line a baking sheet with parchment paper; then, spray the paper with non-stick cooking spray.
- Spread the egg mixture evenly over the parchment paper.
- Bake for 25 minutes. Then remove the cloud bread from heat and set aside.

Ingredients for the Meatball Cloud Bread Sandwich:

- Cloud bread
- Meatballs
- 1 1/3 cups no sugar added tomato sauce
- 2 cups mozzarella cheese

Instructions for the Meatball Cloud Bread Sandwich:

- Prehcat the oven to 350 degrees.
- Cut the cloud bread into four smaller rectangles.
- Place about two meatballs on each rectangle
- Drizzle 1/3 cup no sugar added tomato sauce over each meatball sandwich.
- Sprinkle 1/2 cup of mozzarella over each meatball sandwich.

- Cook in the oven for about 10 minutes or until the cheese is melted
- To eat, gold each rectangle into a "taco" shape and enjoy.

Sweet and Sour Meatballs over Cauliflower Rice

Meatballs are the perfect place to sneak in a little extra nutrients. These meatballs contain dark leafy greens and whole-grain oats, and my children have no idea! Also, remember to look for no sugar added BBQ sauce to keep the sugar content low in this Sweet and Sour Recipe.

Servings: 6

Ingredients for Homemade Meatballs:

- 1 pound lean ground turkey
- 1/2 cup skim milk
- 2 large eggs
- 1/2 package onion soup mix
- 4 oz. frozen spinach
- 1/2 cup uncooked old-fashioned oats
- 1 teaspoon Montreal seasoning
- 1 teaspoon Worcestershire sauce
- 2 teaspoons salt
- 1/2 teaspoon pepper
- Cooking spray

Instructions for the Meatballs:

- Preheat oven to 400 degrees.
- In a medium-mixing bowl, combine all the ingredients except tomato sauce. Line a baking pan with parchment paper.
- Mold your meat into balls using either your hands or a meat baller.

- Bake at 400 degrees for 30-40 minutes or until internal meatball temperature registers 160 degrees.

Ingredients for the Rest of the Recipe:

- 1 onion, cut into slices
- 1 green pepper, cut into slices
- 1 red pepper, cut into slices
- 1 yellow pepper, cut into slices
- 4 cups cauliflower rice (You can use pre-packaged frozen cauliflower rice)
- 2 1/2 cups no sugar added BBQ sauce
- Meatballs from the recipe above

Instructions:

- Add the meatballs and all the other ingredients to the crockpot.
- Cook on "low" setting for 8 hours.

Open-Faced BBQ Chicken and Slaw Sandwich

This is the perfect dinner for those super busy nights. In fact, this dinner requires no cooking! This Easy BBQ Chicken and slaw sandwich contains probiotics, protein, vegetables, and whole-grain bread.

Servings: 4-5

Ingredients:

- 4 cups pre-shredded coleslaw package
- 1/4 cup plain Greek yogurt
- 1/4 cup white cider vinegar
- 1/2 teaspoon garlic powder
- 1 teaspoon yellow mustard seeds
- 1 teaspoon celery seed

- 1/2 teaspoon salt
- 1/2 teaspoon black pepper
- 2, 12.5 ounces cans white meat chicken, drained
- 1 cup BBQ Sauce (I look for no added sugar)
- 1 Tablespoon Hot Sauce (Optional)
- 3-4 whole wheat buns

Instructions:

1. Pour 4 cups of the pre-shredded coleslaw bag into a large bowl.
2. Add the Greek yogurt, white cider vinegar, garlic powder, yellow mustard seeds, celery seeds, salt, and black pepper to the bowl of coleslaw. Mix well with a spoon and set aside.
3. Combine the canned chicken and BBQ sauce in another medium bowl. Add the hot sauce if you like your BBQ spicy. Mix well.
4. Let the chicken marinate in the refrigerator for at least 2 hours or overnight.
5. When you are ready to eat, heat the BBQ in the microwave for approximately 1 minute or until the chicken is warm.
6. Add the BBQ and the slaw to one slice of whole-grain bread. Eat it open-faced like you would a piece of toast.

Greek Yogurt Mayo Open-Faced Turkey Sandwich

Sometimes there is just nothing like a simple sandwich, but this isn't your ordinary turkey sandwich. When your sandwich is topped with guacamole and Italian dressing, every bite is bursting with flavor. Remember to look for no nitrate/nitrite added on the label when you are buying turkey slices.

Serves: 4

Ingredients for the Creamy Ranch Guacamole:

- 2 avocados, peeled and pitted
- 1/3 cup Greek Yogurt, plain
- 1 teaspoon lime or lemon juice
- 2 teaspoon ranch powder
- 1 clove garlic, minced

Instructions for the Creamy Ranch Guacamole:

1. Combine all the ingredients in a medium bowl.
2. Stir and smash the ingredients with a fork or pestle until they are mixed well.
3. Serve with whole-grain chips, crackers, or crispy raw vegetables.

Ingredients for the Sandwich:

- 8 no nitrate/nitrite added turkey slices
- 4 slices provolone cheese
- 8 spinach leaves
- 1 tomato, Sliced
- 4 slices of whole wheat bread
- 4 Tablespoons guacamole
- 4 Tablespoons Italian dressing
- 1 teaspoon black pepper

Instructions for the Sandwich:

- To make this sandwich, spread 1 Tablespoon of guacamole on the slice of bread.
- Then, place the turkey on top of a slice of whole-grain bread.
- Next, add a piece of provolone cheese and a slice of tomato. Top the cheese with a couple of spinach leaves.
- Drizzle the spinach leaves with Italian dressing.
- Then sprinkle a pinch of black pepper.
- Do these steps for 4 open-faced sandwiches.

Black Bean Soup

Finally, I couldn't end this collection of delicious recipes without adding this comforting warm Black Bean soup. It's plant-based and a great source of protein and antioxidants. Top it with tortilla chips and avocado to add flavor and crunch.

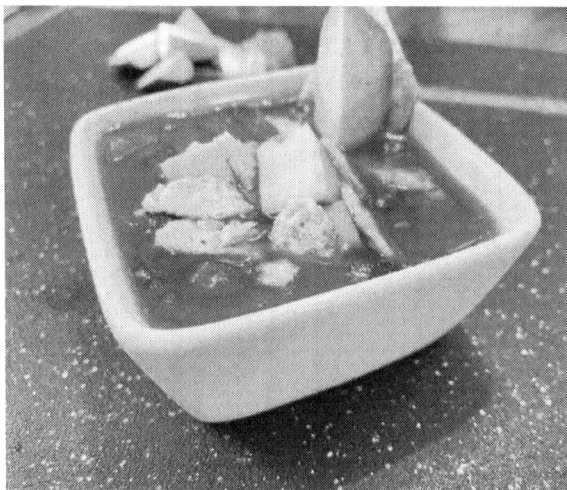

Serves: 8

Ingredients:

- 3 cups canned black beans, drained
- 2 cups canned tomato soup
- 1 onion, chopped
- 1 cup vegetable broth
- 1/2 cup cilantro leaves (leave a few out for a garnish)
- 4 cloves garlic, minced
- 1 Tablespoon lime juice
- 2 Tablespoons taco seasoning
- 1 avocado, peeled and sliced
- Optional light sour cream and tortilla chips (I look for whole grain, bean, or sced tortilla chips)

Instructions:

- Add all the ingredients except the avocado slices into a large pot.
- Bring the soup to a boil, then reduce the heat to low.
- Cover and simmer for about 20 minutes.
- Serve the soup topped with avocado slices. You can also add broken-up tortilla chips and/or a dollop of light sour cream.

References

1. Addolorato, G., Marsigli, L., Capristo, E., Caputo, F., Dall'Aglio, C., & Baudanza, P. (1998). Anxiety and depression: a common feature of health care seeking patients with irritable bowel syndrome and food allergy. *Hepato-Gastroenterology*, 45(23), 1559–1564. **http://europepmc.org/article/med/9840105**

2. Akbari, E., Asemi, Z., Daneshvar Kakhaki, R., Bahmani, F., Kouchaki, E., Tamtaji, O. R., Hamidi, G. A., & Salami, M. (2016). Effect of Probiotic Supplementation on Cognitive Function and Metabolic Status in Alzheimer's Disease: A Randomized, Double-Blind and Controlled Trial. *Frontiers in Aging Neuroscience*, 8. https://doi.org/**10.3389/fnagi.2016.00256**

3. Akhondzadeh, S., Noroozian, M., Mohammadi, M., Ohadinia, S., Jamshidi, A. H., & Khani, M. (2003). Salvia officinalis extract in the treatment of patients with mild to moderate Alzheimer's disease: a double blind, randomized and placebo-controlled trial. *Journal of Clinical Pharmacy and Therapeutics*, 28(1), 53–59. https://doi.org/**10.1046/j.1365-2710.2003.00463.x**

4. Akkasheh, G., Kashani-Poor, Z., Tajabadi-Ebrahimi, M., Jafari, P., Akbari, H., Taghizadeh, M., Memarzadeh, M. R., Asemi, Z., & Esmaillzadeh, A. (2016). Clinical and metabolic response to probiotic administration in patients with major depressive disorder: A randomized, double-blind, placebo-controlled trial. *Nutrition*, 32(3), 315–320. https://doi.org/**10.1016/j.nut.2015.09.003**

5. Amalraj, A., Pius, A., Gopi, S., & Gopi, S. (2017). Biological activities of curcuminoids, other biomolecules from turmeric and their derivatives – A review. *Journal of Traditional and Complementary Medicine*, 7(2), 205–233. https://doi.org/**10.1016/j.jtcme.2016.05.005**

6. Andrade, J. M., Faustino, C., Garcia, C., Ladeiras, D., Reis, C. P., & Rijo, P. (2018). Rosmarinus officinalis L.: an update review of its phytochemistry and biological activity. *Future Science OA*, 4(4), FSO283. https://doi.org/**10.4155/fsoa-2017-0124**

7. Andrade, S., Ramalho, M. J., Pereira, M. do C., & Loureiro, J. A. (2018). Resveratrol Brain Delivery for Neurological Disorders Prevention and Treatment. *Frontiers in Pharmacology*, 9. https://doi.org/**10.3389/fphar.2018.01261**

8. Anghelescu, I.-G., Edwards, D., Seifritz, E., & Kasper, S. (2018). Stress management and the role of Rhodiola rosea: a review. *International Journal of Psychiatry in Clinical Practice*, 22(4), 242–252. https://doi.org/**10.1080/13651501.2017.1417442**

9. Appelhans, B. M., Whited, M. C., Schneider, K. L., Ma, Y., Oleski, J. L., Merriam, P. A., Waring, M. E., Olendzki, B. C., Mann, D. M., Ockene, I. S., & Pagoto, S. L. (2012). Depression Severity, Diet Quality, and Physical Activity in Women with Obesity and Depression. *Journal of the Academy of Nutrition and Dietetics*, 112(5), 693–698. https://doi.org/**10.1016/j.jand.2012.02.006**

10. Ballmann, C. G., Maze, S. B., Wells, A. C., Marshall, M. R., & Rogers, R. R. (2018). Effects of short-term Rhodiola Rosea (Golden Root Extract) supplementation on anaerobic exercise performance. *Journal of Sports Sciences*, *37*(9), 998–1003. https://doi.org/**10.1080/02640414.2018.1538028**

11. Banjari, I., Vukoje, I., & Mandic, M. L. (2014). *(PDF) BRAIN FOOD: HOW NUTRITION ALTERS OUR MOOD AND BEHAVIOUR.* ResearchGate. ***https://www.researchgate.net/publication/263620765 BRAIN FOOD HOW NUTRITION ALTERS OUR MOOD AND BEHAVIOUR***

12. Bauer, M. E., & Teixeira, A. L. (2018). Inflammation in psychiatric disorders: what comes first? *Annals of the New York Academy of Sciences*, *1437*(1), 57–67. https://doi.org/**10.1111/nyas.13712**

13. Bianchi, V. E., Herrera, P. F., & Laura, R. (2019). Effect of nutrition on neurodegenerative diseases. A systematic review. *Nutritional Neuroscience*, 1–25. https://doi.org/**10.1080/1028415x.2019.1681088**

14. Blacher, E., Bashiardes, S., Shapiro, H., Rothschild, D., Mor, U., Dori-Bachash, M., Kleimeyer, C., Moresi, C., Harnik, Y., Zur, M., Zabari, M., Brik, R. B.-Z., Kviatcovsky, D., Zmora, N., Cohen, Y., Bar, N., Levi, I., Amar, N., Mehlman, T., & Brandis, A. (2019). Potential roles of gut microbiome and metabolites in modulating ALS in mice. *Nature*, *572*(7770), 474–480. https://doi.org/**10.1038/s41586-019-1443-5**

15. Black, C. D., Herring, M. P., Hurley, D. J., & O'Connor, P. J. (2010). Ginger (Zingiber officinale) Reduces Muscle Pain Caused by Eccentric Exercise. *The Journal of Pain*, *11*(9), 894–903. https://doi.org/**10.1016/j.jpain.2009.12.013**

16. Boyer, J., & Liu, R. H. (2004). Apple phytochemicals and their health benefits. *Nutrition Journal*, *3*(1). https://doi.org/**10.1186/1475-2891-3-5**

17. Braga, V. L., Rocha, L. P. D. S., Bernardo, D. D., Cruz, C. de O., & Riera, R. (2017). What do Cochrane systematic reviews say about probiotics as preventive interventions? *Sao Paulo Medical Journal = Revista Paulista de Medicina*, *135*(6), 578–586. https://doi.org/**10.1590/1516-3180.2017.0310241017**

18. Cannell, J. J., & Hollis, B. W. (2008). Use of vitamin D in clinical practice. *Alternative Medicine Review: A Journal of Clinical Therapeutic*, *13*(1), 6–20. ***https://pubmed.ncbi.nlm.nih.gov/18377099/***

19. Carroll, R. E., Benya, R. V., Turgeon, D. K., Vareed, S., Neuman, M., Rodriguez, L., Kakarala, M., Carpenter, P. M., McLaren, C., Meyskens, F. L., & Brenner, D. E. (2011). Phase IIa Clinical Trial of Curcumin for the Prevention of Colorectal Neoplasia. *Cancer Prevention Research*, *4*(3), 354–364. https://doi.org/**10.1158/1940-6207.capr-10-0098**

20. Chang, J. S., Wang, K. C., Yeh, C. F., Shieh, D. E., & Chiang, L. C. (2013). Fresh ginger (Zingiber officinale) has anti-viral activity against human respiratory syncytial virus in human respiratory tract cell lines. *Journal*

of *Ethnopharmacology*, *145*(1), 146–151. https://doi.org/**10.1016/j.jep.2012.10.043**

21. Chen, X., Huang, Y., & Cheng, H. G. (2012). Lower intake of vegetables and legumes associated with cognitive decline among illiterate elderly Chinese: a 3-year cohort study. *The Journal of Nutrition, Health & Aging*, *16*(6), 549–552. https://doi.org/**10.1007/s12603-012-0023-2**

22. Choi, F. D., Sung, C. T., Juhasz, M. L. W., & Mesinkovsk, N. A. (2019). Oral Collagen Supplementation: A Systematic Review of Dermatological Applications. *Journal of Drugs in Dermatology: JDD*, *18*(1), 9–16. ***https://pubmed.ncbi.nlm.nih.gov/30681787/***

23. Chunchai, T., Thunapong, W., Yasom, S., Wanchai, K., Eaimworawuthikul, S., Metzler, G., Lungkaphin, A., Pongchaidecha, A., Sirilun, S., Chaiyasut, C., Pratchayasakul, W., Thiennimitr, P., Chattipakorn, N., & Chattipakorn, S. C. (2018). Decreased microglial activation through gut-brain axis by prebiotics, probiotics, or synbiotics effectively restored cognitive function in obese-insulin resistant rats. *Journal of Neuroinflammation*, *15*, 11. https://doi.org/**10.1186/s12974-018-1055-2**

24. Curtis L;Epstein P. (2014). Nutritional treatment for acute and chronic traumatic brain injury patients. *Journal of Neurosurgical Sciences*, *58*(3). ***https://pubmed.ncbi.nlm.nih.gov/24844176/***

25. Das, R. R., Singh, M., & Shafiq, N. (2010). Probiotics for Prevention or Treatment of Asthma. *Chest*, *138*(4), 307A. https://doi.org/**10.1378/chest.9485**

26. Davari, S., Talaei, S. A., Alaei, H., & salami, M. (2013). Probiotics treatment improves diabetes-induced impairment of synaptic activity and cognitive function: Behavioral and electrophysiological proofs for microbiome–gut–brain axis. *Neuroscience*, *240*, 287–296. https://doi.org/**10.1016/j.neuroscience.2013.02.055**

27. Fata, G., Weber, P., & Mohajeri, M. (2014). Effects of Vitamin E on Cognitive Performance during Ageing and in Alzheimer's Disease. *Nutrients*, *6*(12), 5453–5472. https://doi.org/**10.3390/nu6125453**

28. Fedoreyev, S. A., Krylova, N. V., Mishchenko, N. P., Vasileva, E. A., Pislyagin, E. A., Iunikhina, O. V., Lavrov, V. F., Svitich, O. A., Ebralidze, L. K., & Leonova, G. N. (2018). Antiviral and Antioxidant Properties of Echinochrome A. *Marine Drugs*, *16*(12), 509. https://doi.org/**10.3390/md16120509**

29. Fitzgerald, K. C., O'Reilly, É. J., Fondell, E., Falcone, G. J., McCullough, M. L., Park, Y., Kolonel, L. N., & Ascherio, A. (2013). Intakes of vitamin C and carotenoids and risk of amyotrophic lateral sclerosis: Pooled results from 5 cohort studies. *Annals of Neurology*, *73*(2), 236–245. https://doi.org/**10.1002/ana.23820**

30. Furushima, D., Ide, K., & Yamada, H. (2018). Effect of Tea Catechins on Influenza Infection and the Common Cold with a Focus on Epidemiological/Clinical Studies. *Molecules*, *23*(7), 1795. https://doi.org/**10.3390/molecules23071795**

31. Gautam, M., Agrawal, M., Gautam, M., Sharma, P., Gautam, A., & Gautam, S. (2012). Role of antioxidants in generalised anxiety disorder and depression. *Indian Journal of Psychiatry*, *54*(3), 244. https://doi.org/**10.4103/0019-5545.102424**

32. Gómez-Pinilla, F. (2008). Brain foods: the effects of nutrients on brain function. *Nature Reviews Neuroscience*, *9*(7), 568–578. https://doi.org/**10.1038/nrn2421**

33. Griffin, R. M. (2010). *Natural Cold and Flu Remedies*. WebMD. **https://www.webmd.com/a-to-z-guides/features/colds-flu-immune-system#1**

34. Guilleminault, L., Williams, E., Scott, H., Berthon, B., Jensen, M., & Wood, L. (2017). Diet and Asthma: Is It Time to Adapt Our Message? *Nutrients*, *9*(11), 1227. https://doi.org/**10.3390/nu9111227**

35. Guzmán, J. F., Esteve, H., Pablos, C., Pablos, A., Blasco, C., & Villegas, J. A. (2011). DHA- Rich Fish Oil Improves Complex Reaction Time in Female Elite Soccer Players. *Journal of Sports Science & Medicine*, *10*(2), 301–305. **https://pubmed.ncbi.nlm.nih.gov/24149875/**

36. Habtemariam, S. (2016). The Therapeutic Potential of Rosemary (Rosmarinus officinalis) Diterpenes for Alzheimer's Disease. *Evidence-Based Complementary and Alternative Medicine*, *2016*, 1–14. https://doi.org/**10.1155/2016/2680409**

37. Hansen, A., Olson, G., Dahl, L., Thornton, D., Grung, B., Graff, I., Frøyland, L., & Thayer, J. (2014). Reduced Anxiety in Forensic Inpatients after a Long-Term Intervention with Atlantic Salmon. *Nutrients*, *6*(12), 5405–5418. https://doi.org/**10.3390/nu6125405**

38. Hardman, W. E. (2014). Walnuts Have Potential for Cancer Prevention and Treatment in Mice. *The Journal of Nutrition*, *144*(4), 555S560S. https://doi.org/**10.3945/jn.113.188466**

39. Harms, L. R., Burne, T. H. J., Eyles, D. W., & McGrath, J. J. (2011). Vitamin D and the brain. *Best Practice & Research Clinical Endocrinology & Metabolism*, *25*(4), 657–669. https://doi.org/**10.1016/j.beem.2011.05.009**

40. Harri, H. (2011). Zinc Lozenges May Shorten the Duration of Colds: A Systematic Review. *The Open Respiratory Medicine Journal*, *5*(1), 51–58. https://doi.org/**10.2174/1874306401105010051**

41. Hasadsri, L., Wang, B. H., Lee, J. V., Erdman, J. W., Llano, D. A., Barbey, A. K., Wszalek, T., Sharrock, M. F., & Wang, H. J. (2013). Omega-3 fatty acids as a putative treatment for traumatic brain injury. *Journal of Neurotrauma*, *30*(11), 897–906. https://doi.org/**10.1089/neu.2012.2672**

42. Hemilä, H., & Chalker, E. (2013). Vitamin C for preventing and treating the common cold. *Cochrane Database of Systematic Reviews*. https://doi.org/**10.1002/14651858.cd000980.pub4**

43. Hersi, M., Irvine, B., Gupta, P., Gomes, J., Birkett, N., & Krewski, D. (2017). Risk factors associated with the onset and progression of Alzheimer's disease: A systematic review of the evidence.

NeuroToxicology, 61, 143–187.
https://doi.org/**10.1016/j.neuro.2017.03.006**

44. Hirsch, K., Danilenko, M., Giat, J., Miron, T., Rabinkov, A., Wilchek, M., Mirelman, D., Levy, J., & Sharoni, Y. (2000). Effect of Purified Allicin, the Major Ingredient ofFreshly Crushed Garlic, on Cancer Cell Proliferation. *Nutrition and Cancer, 38*(2), 245–254.
https://doi.org/**10.1207/s15327914nc382_14**

45. Howatson, G., Bell, P. G., Tallent, J., Middleton, B., McHugh, M. P., & Ellis, J. (2011). Effect of tart cherry juice (Prunus cerasus) on melatonin levels and enhanced sleep quality. *European Journal of Nutrition, 51*(8), 909–916. https://doi.org/**10.1007/s00394-011-0263-7**

46. Hu, P., Bretsky, P., Crimmins, E. M., Guralnik, J. M., Reuben, D. B., & Seeman, T. E. (2006). Association Between Serum Beta-Carotene Levels and Decline of Cognitive Function in High-Functioning Older Persons With or Without Apolipoprotein E 4 Alleles: MacArthur Studies of Successful Aging. *The Journals of Gerontology Series A: Biological Sciences and Medical Sciences, 61*(6), 616–620.
https://doi.org/**10.1093/gerona/61.6.616**

47. Huang, Q., Liu, H., Suzuki, K., Ma, S., & Liu, C. (2019). Linking What We Eat to Our Mood: A Review of Diet, Dietary Antioxidants, and Depression. *Antioxidants, 8*(9), 376.
https://doi.org/**10.3390/antiox8090376**

48. Huang, R., Wang, K., & Hu, J. (2016). Effect of Probiotics on Depression: A Systematic Review and Meta-Analysis of Randomized Controlled Trials. *Nutrients, 8*(8), 483. https://doi.org/**10.3390/nu8080483**

49. Jamshidi, N., & Cohen, M. M. (2017). The Clinical Efficacy and Safety of Tulsi in Humans: A Systematic Review of the Literature. *Evidence-Based Complementary and Alternative Medicine : ECAM, 2017.*
https://doi.org/**10.1155/2017/9217567**

50. Janssens, P. L. H. R., Hursel, R., Martens, E. A. P., & Westerterp-Plantenga, M. S. (2013). Acute Effects of Capsaicin on Energy Expenditure and Fat Oxidation in Negative Energy Balance. *PLoS ONE, 8*(7), e67786. https://doi.org/**10.1371/journal.pone.0067786**

51. Jia, K., Tong, X., Wang, R., & Song, X. (2018). The clinical effects of probiotics for inflammatory bowel disease. *Medicine, 97*(51).
https://doi.org/**10.1097/MD.0000000000013792**

52. Johnson, E. J., Mcdonald, K., Caldarella, S. M., Chung, H., Troen, A. M., & Snodderly, D. M. (2008). Cognitive findings of an exploratory trial of docosahexaenoic acid and lutein supplementation in older women. *Nutritional Neuroscience, 11*(2), 75–83.
https://doi.org/**10.1179/147683008x301450**

53. Kalt, W., Cassidy, A., Howard, L. R., Krikorian, R., Stull, A. J., Tremblay, F., & Zamora-Ros, R. (2019). Recent research on the health benefits of blueberries and their anthocyanins. *Advances in Nutrition, 11*(2).
https://doi.org/**10.1093/advances/nmz065**

54. Kanauchi, O., Andoh, A., AbuBakar, S., & Yamamoto, N. (2018). Probiotics and Paraprobiotics in Viral Infection: Clinical Application and Effects on the Innate and Acquired Immune Systems. *Current*

Pharmaceutical Design, 24(6), 710–717.
https://doi.org/**10.2174/1381612824666180116163411**

55. Kang, E.-J., Kim, S. Y., Hwang, I.-H., & Ji, Y.-J. (2013). The Effect of Probiotics on Prevention of Common Cold: A Meta-Analysis of Randomized Controlled Trial Studies. *Korean Journal of Family Medicine, 34*(1), 2. https://doi.org/**10.4082/kjfm.2013.34.1.2**

56. Katz Sand, I. (2018). The Role of Diet in Multiple Sclerosis: Mechanistic Connections and Current Evidence. *Current Nutrition Reports, 7*(3), 150–160. https://doi.org/**10.1007/s13668-018-0236-z**

57. Kiecolt-Glaser, J. K., Derry, H. M., & Fagundes, C. P. (2015). Inflammation: Depression Fans the Flames and Feasts on the Heat. *American Journal of Psychiatry, 172*(11), 1075–1091. https://doi.org/**10.1176/appi.ajp.2015.15020152**

58. King, S., Glanville, J., Sanders, M. E., Fitzgerald, A., & Varley, D. (2014). Effectiveness of probiotics on the duration of illness in healthy children and adults who develop common acute respiratory infectious conditions: a systematic review and meta-analysis. *British Journal of Nutrition, 112*(1), 41–54. https://doi.org/**10.1017/S0007114514000075**

59. Kontush, K., & Schekatolina, S. (2004). Vitamin E in neurodegenerative disorders: Alzheimer's disease. *Annals of the New York Academy of Sciences, 1031*, 249–262. https://doi.org/**10.1196/annals.1331.025**

60. Kreider, R. B., Kalman, D. S., Antonio, J., Ziegenfuss, T. N., Wildman, R., Collins, R., Candow, D. G., Kleiner, S. M., Almada, A. L., & Lopez, H. L. (2017). International Society of Sports Nutrition position stand: safety and efficacy of creatine supplementation in exercise, sport, and medicine. *Journal of the International Society of Sports Nutrition, 14*(1). https://doi.org/**10.1186/s12970-017-0173-z**

61. Kresty, L. A., Morse, M. A., Morgan, C., Carlton, P. S., Lu, J., Gupta, A., Blackwood, M., & Stoner, G. D. (2001). Chemoprevention of esophageal tumorigenesis by dietary administration of lyophilized black raspberries. *Cancer Research, 61*(16), 6112–6119. ***https://pubmed.ncbi.nlm.nih.gov/11507061/***

62. Krylova, N. V., Popov, A. M., & Leonova, G. N. (2016). Antioxidants as Potential Antiviral Agents for Flavivirus Infections. *Antibiotiki I Khimioterapiia = Antibiotics and Chemoterapy [Sic], 61*(5-6), 25–31. ***https://pubmed.ncbi.nlm.nih.gov/29537738/***

63. Krysiak, R., Szkróbka, W., & Okopień, B. (2018). The Effect of Gluten-Free Diet on Thyroid Autoimmunity in Drug-Naïve Women with Hashimoto's Thyroiditis: A Pilot Study. *Experimental and Clinical Endocrinology & Diabetes, 127*(07), 417–422. https://doi.org/**10.1055/a-0653-7108**

64. Kwon, H.-K., Hwang, J.-S., So, J.-S., Lee, C.-G., Sahoo, A., Ryu, J.-H., Jeon, W. K., Ko, B. S., Im, C.-R., Lee, S. H., Park, Z. Y., & Im, S.-H. (2010). Cinnamon extract induces tumor cell death through inhibition of NFκB and AP1. *BMC Cancer, 10*(1). https://doi.org/**10.1186/1471-2407-10-392**

65. Lang, U. E., Beglinger, C., Schweinfurth, N., Walter, M., & Borgwardt, S. (2015). Nutritional Aspects of Depression. *Cellular Physiology and*

Biochemistry, 37(3), 1029–1043.
https://doi.org/**10.1159/000430229**

66. Laursen, R. P., & Hojsak, I. (2018). Probiotics for respiratory tract infections in children attending day care centers—a systematic review. *European Journal of Pediatrics, 177*(7), 979–994. https://doi.org/**10.1007/s00431-018-3167-1**

67. Lehtoranta, L., Pitkäranta, A., & Korpela, R. (2014). Probiotics in respiratory virus infections. *European Journal of Clinical Microbiology & Infectious Diseases, 33*(8), 1289–1302. https://doi.org/**10.1007/s10096-014-2086-y**

68. Li, Y., Lv, M.-R., Wei, Y.-J., Sun, L., Zhang, J.-X., Zhang, H.-G., & Li, B. (2017). Dietary patterns and depression risk: A meta-analysis. *Psychiatry Research, 253*, 373–382. https://doi.org/**10.1016/j.psychres.2017.04.020**

69. Li, Y., Zhang, T., Korkaya, H., Liu, S., Lee, H. F., Newman, B., Yu, Y., Clouthier, S. G., Schwartz, S. J., Wicha, M. S., & Sun, D. (2010). Sulforaphane, a Dietary Component of Broccoli/Broccoli Sprouts, Inhibits Breast Cancer Stem Cells. *Clinical Cancer Research, 16*(9), 2580–2590. https://doi.org/**10.1158/1078-0432.ccr-09-2937**

70. Lissiman, E., Bhasale, A., & Cohen, M. (2020). *Garlic for the common cold.* Www.cochrane.org.
https://www.cochrane.org/CD006206/ARI_garlic-common-cold

71. Liu, Y., Alookaran, J., & Rhoads, J. (2018). Probiotics in Autoimmune and Inflammatory Disorders. *Nutrients, 10*(10), 1537. https://doi.org/**10.3390/nu10101537**

72. Lopresti, A. L., Smith, S. J., Malvi, H., & Kodgule, R. (2019). An investigation into the stress-relieving and pharmacological actions of an ashwagandha (Withania somnifera) extract: A randomized, double-blind, placebo-controlled study. *Medicine, 98*(37), e17186. https://doi.org/**10.1097/MD.0000000000017186**

73. Manzel, A., Muller, D. N., Hafler, D. A., Erdman, S. E., Linker, R. A., & Kleinewietfeld, M. (2013). Role of "Western Diet" in Inflammatory Autoimmune Diseases. *Current Allergy and Asthma Reports, 14*(1). https://doi.org/**10.1007/s11882-013-0404-6**

74. Martínez García, R. M., Jiménez Ortega, A. I., López Sobaler, A. M., & Ortega Anta, R. M. (2018). Estrategias nutricionales que mejoran la función cognitiva. *Nutrición Hospitalaria, 35*(6). https://doi.org/**10.20960/nh.2281**

75. Martínez-Lapiscina, E. H., Clavero, P., Toledo, E., Estruch, R., Salas-Salvadó, J., San Julián, B., Sanchez-Tainta, A., Ros, E., Valls-Pedret, C., & Martinez-Gonzalez, M. Á. (2013). Mediterranean diet improves cognition: the PREDIMED-NAVARRA randomised trial. *Journal of Neurology, Neurosurgery & Psychiatry, 84*(12), 1318–1325. https://doi.org/**10.1136/jnnp-2012-304792**

76. Matheson, E. M., King, D. E., & Everett, C. J. (2012). Healthy lifestyle habits and mortality in overweight and obese individuals. *Journal of the*

American Board of Family Medicine : JABFM, 25(1), 9–15. https://doi.org/**10.3122/jabfm.2012.01.110164**

77. Mazzini, L., Mogna, L., De Marchi, F., Amoruso, A., Pane, M., Aloisio, I., Cionci, N. B., Gaggìa, F., Lucenti, A., Bersano, E., Cantello, R., Di Gioia, D., & Mogna, G. (2018). Potential Role of Gut Microbiota in ALS Pathogenesis and Possible Novel Therapeutic Strategies. *Journal of Clinical Gastroenterology, 52 Suppl 1, Proceedings from the 9th Probiotics, Prebiotics and New Foods, Nutraceuticals and Botanicals for Nutrition & Human and Microbiota Health Meeting, held in Rome, Italy from September 10 to 12, 2017*, S68–S70. https://doi.org/**10.1097/MCG.0000000000001042**

78. Mentella, Scaldaferri, Ricci, Gasbarrini, & Miggiano. (2019). Cancer and Mediterranean Diet: A Review. *Nutrients, 11*(9), 2059. https://doi.org/**10.3390/nu11092059**

79. Messaoudi, M., Lalonde, R., Violle, N., Javelot, H., Desor, D., Nejdi, A., Bisson, J.-F., Rougeot, C., Pichelin, M., Cazaubiel, M., & Cazaubiel, J.-M. (2010). Assessment of psychotropic-like properties of a probiotic formulation (Lactobacillus helveticus R0052 and Bifidobacterium longum R0175) in rats and human subjects. *British Journal of Nutrition, 105*(5), 755–764. https://doi.org/**10.1017/S0007114510004319**

80. Miki, T., Eguchi, M., Kurotani, K., Kochi, T., Kuwahara, K., Ito, R., Kimura, Y., Tsuruoka, H., Akter, S., Kashino, I., Kabe, I., Kawakami, N., & Mizoue, T. (2016). Dietary fiber intake and depressive symptoms in Japanese employees: The Furukawa Nutrition and Health Study. *Nutrition, 32*(5), 584–589. https://doi.org/**10.1016/j.nut.2015.11.014**

81. Miller, M. G., Hamilton, D. A., Joseph, J. A., & Shukitt-Hale, B. (2018). Dietary blueberry improves cognition among older adults in a randomized, double-blind, placebo-controlled trial. *European Journal of Nutrition, 57*(3), 1169–1180. https://doi.org/**10.1007/s00394-017-1400-8**

82. Miyata, J., & Arita, M. (2015). Role of omega-3 fatty acids and their metabolites in asthma and allergic diseases. *Allergology International: Official Journal of the Japanese Society of Allergology, 64*(1), 27–34. https://doi.org/**10.1016/j.alit.2014.08.003**

83. Mohammadi, A. A., Jazayeri, S., Khosravi-Darani, K., Solati, Z., Mohammadpour, N., Asemi, Z., Adab, Z., Djalali, M., Tehrani-Doost, M., Hosseini, M., & Eghtesadi, S. (2015). The effects of probiotics on mental health and hypothalamic–pituitary–adrenal axis: A randomized, double-blind, placebo-controlled trial in petrochemical workers. *Nutritional Neuroscience, 19*(9), 387–395. https://doi.org/**10.1179/1476830515y.0000000023**

84. Mora, J. R., Iwata, M., & von Andrian, U. H. (2008). Vitamin effects on the immune system: vitamins A and D take centre stage. *Nature Reviews Immunology, 8*(9), 685–698. https://doi.org/**10.1038/nri2378**

85. Morris, M. C. (2011). Nutritional determinants of cognitive aging and dementia. *Proceedings of the Nutrition Society, 71*(1), 1–13. https://doi.org/**10.1017/s0029665111003296**

86. Morris, M. C., Tangney, C. C., Wang, Y., Sacks, F. M., Barnes, L. L., Bennett, D. A., & Aggarwal, N. T. (2015). MIND diet slows cognitive decline with aging. *Alzheimer's & Dementia, 11*(9), 1015–1022. https://doi.org/**10.1016/j.jalz.2015.04.011**

87. Muhammad, D. R. A., & Dewettinck, K. (2017). Cinnamon and its derivatives as potential ingredient in functional food—A review. *International Journal of Food Properties, 1–27.* https://doi.org/**10.1080/10942912.2017.1369102**

88. MUJIKA, I., PADILLA, S., IBA??EZ, J., IZQUIERDO, M., & GOROSTIAGA, E. (2000). Creatine supplementation and sprint performance in soccer players. *Medicine & Science in Sports & Exercise, 32*(2), 518. https://doi.org/**10.1097/00005768-200002000-00039**

89. Munger, K. L., & Ascherio, A. (2011). Prevention and treatment of MS: studying the effects of vitamin D. *Multiple Sclerosis (Houndmills, Basingstoke, England), 17*(12), 1405. https://doi.org/**10.1177/1352458511425366**

90. Nair, A., Amalraj, A., Jacob, J., Kunnumakkara, A. B., & Gopi, S. (2019). Non-Curcuminoids from Turmeric and Their Potential in Cancer Therapy and Anticancer Drug Delivery Formulations. *Biomolecules, 9*(1), 13. https://doi.org/**10.3390/biom9010013**

91. Nantz, M. P., Rowe, C. A., Muller, C., Creasy, R., Colee, J., Khoo, C., & Percival, S. S. (2013). Consumption of cranberry polyphenols enhances human γδ-T cell proliferation and reduces the number of symptoms associated with colds and influenza: a randomized, placebo-controlled intervention study. *Nutrition Journal, 12*(1). https://doi.org/**10.1186/1475-2891-12-161**

92. National Center for Complementary and Integrative Health. (2019, August). *Probiotics: What You Need To Know*. NCCIH. **https://www.nccih.nih.gov/health/probiotics-what-you-need-to-know**

93. National Institute on Aging. (2019, November 30). What Do We Know About Diet and Prevention of Alzheimer's Disease? *National Institutes of Health.* **https://www.nia.nih.gov/health/what-do-we-know-about-diet-and-prevention-alzheimers-disease**

94. Nazir, Y., Hussain, S. A., Abdul Hamid, A., & Song, Y. (2018). Probiotics and Their Potential Preventive and Therapeutic Role for Cancer, High Serum Cholesterol, and Allergic and HIV Diseases. *BioMed Research International, 2018*, 1–17. https://doi.org/**10.1155/2018/3428437**

95. NIEMAN, D. C., HENSON, D. A., GROSS, S. J., JENKINS, D. P., DAVIS, J. M., MURPHY, E. A., CARMICHAEL, M. D., DUMKE, C. L., UTTER, A. C., MCANULTY, S. R., MCANULTY, L. S., & MAYER, E. P. (2007). Quercetin Reduces Illness but Not Immune Perturbations after Intensive Exercise. *Medicine & Science in Sports & Exercise, 39*(9), 1561–1569. https://doi.org/**10.1249/mss.0b013e318076b566**

96. O'Neil, A., Quirk, S. E., Housden, S., Brennan, S. L., Williams, L. J., Pasco, J. A., Berk, M., & Jacka, F. N. (2014). Relationship Between Diet and Mental Health in Children and Adolescents: A Systematic Review.

American Journal of Public Health, 104(10), e31–e42.
https://doi.org/**10.2105/ajph.2014.302110**

97. Oommen, S., Anto, R. J., Srinivas, G., & Karunagaran, D. (2004). Allicin (from garlic) induces caspase-mediated apoptosis in cancer cells. *European Journal of Pharmacology, 485*(1-3), 97–103.
https://doi.org/**10.1016/j.ejphar.2003.11.059**

98. Palmer, S. (2011). *Is There a Link Between Nutrition and Autoimmune Disease?* Www.todaysdietitian.com.
***https://www.todaysdietitian.com/newarchives/110211p
36.shtml***

99. Parisi, A., Tranchita, E., Duranti, G., Ciminelli, E., Quaranta, F., Ceci, R., Cerulli, C., Borrione, P., & Sabatini, S. (2010). Effects of chronic Rhodiola Rosea supplementation on sport performance and antioxidant capacity in trained male: preliminary results. *The Journal of Sports Medicine and Physical Fitness, 50*(1), 57–63.
***https://pubmed.ncbi.nlm.nih.gov/20308973/#:~:text=M
ethods%3A%20Following%20a%20chronic%20supplem
entation%20with%20Rhodiola%20Rosea***

100. Payne, M. E., Steck, S. E., George, R. R., & Steffens, D. C. (2012). Fruit, vegetable, and antioxidant intakes are lower in older adults with depression. *Journal of the Academy of Nutrition and Dietetics, 112*(12), 2022–2027. https://doi.org/**10.1016/j.jand.2012.08.026**

101. Pengelly, A., Snow, J., Mills, S. Y., Scholey, A., Wesnes, K., & Butler, L. R. (2012). Short-term study on the effects of rosemary on cognitive function in an elderly population. *Journal of Medicinal Food, 15*(1), 10–17.
https://doi.org/**10.1089/jmf.2011.0005**

102. Pérez-Gómez, J., Villafaina, S., Adsuar, J. C., Merellano-Navarro, E., & Collado-Mateo, D. (2020). Effects of Ashwagandha (Withania somnifera) on VO2max: A Systematic Review and Meta-Analysis. *Nutrients, 12*(4), 1119. https://doi.org/**10.3390/nu12041119**

103. Petersson, S., Philippou, E., Rodomar, C., & Nikiphorou, E. (2018). The Mediterranean diet, fish oil supplements and Rheumatoid arthritis outcomes: evidence from clinical trials. *Autoimmunity Reviews, 17*(11), 1105–1114. https://doi.org/**10.1016/j.autrev.2018.06.007**

104. Pham, N. M., Nanri, A., Kurotani, K., Kuwahara, K., Kume, A., Sato, M., Hayabuchi, H., & Mizoue, T. (2013). Green tea and coffee consumption is inversely associated with depressive symptoms in a Japanese working population. *Public Health Nutrition, 17*(3), 625–633.
https://doi.org/**10.1017/s1368980013000360**

105. Ptomey, L. T., Steger, F. L., Schubert, M. M., Lee, J., Willis, E. A., Sullivan, D. K., Szabo-Reed, A. N., Washburn, R. A., & Donnelly, J. E. (2015). Breakfast Intake and Composition Is Associated with Superior Academic Achievement in Elementary Schoolchildren. *Journal of the American College of Nutrition, 35*(4), 326–333.
https://doi.org/**10.1080/07315724.2015.1048381**

106. Research, F. A. B. (2017). *FAB: Amen et al 2017 - Quantitative Erythrocyte Omega-3 EPA Plus DHA Levels are Related to Higher*

Regional Cerebral Blood Flow on Brain SPECT. Www.fabresearch.org.
https://www.fabresearch.org/viewItem.php?id=10965

107.   Rizvi, S., Raza, S. T., Ahmed, F., Ahmad, A., Abbas, S., & Mahdi, F. (2014). The role of vitamin e in human health and some diseases. *Sultan Qaboos University Medical Journal*, *14*(2), e157-165. ***https://pubmed.ncbi.nlm.nih.gov/24790736/***

108.   Roman, P., Estévez, A. F., Miras, A., Sánchez-Labraca, N., Cañadas, F., Vivas, A. B., & Cardona, D. (2018). A Pilot Randomized Controlled Trial to Explore Cognitive and Emotional Effects of Probiotics in Fibromyalgia. *Scientific Reports*, *8*(1). https://doi.org/***10.1038/s41598-018-29388-5***

109.   Rondanelli, M., Miccono, A., Lamburghini, S., Avanzato, I., Riva, A., Allegrini, P., Faliva, M. A., Peroni, G., Nichetti, M., & Perna, S. (2018). Self-Care for Common Colds: The Pivotal Role of Vitamin D, Vitamin C, Zinc, and Echinacea in Three Main Immune Interactive Clusters (Physical Barriers, Innate and Adaptive Immunity) Involved during an Episode of Common Colds—Practical Advice on Dosages and on the Time to Take These Nutrients/Botanicals in order to Prevent or Treat Common Colds. *Evidence-Based Complementary and Alternative Medicine*, *2018*, 1–36. https://doi.org/***10.1155/2018/5813095***

110. Saghafian, F., Malmir, H., Saneei, P., Milajerdi, A., Larijani, B., & Esmaillzadeh, A. (2018). Fruit and vegetable consumption and risk of depression: accumulative evidence from an updated systematic review and meta-analysis of epidemiological studies. *The British Journal of Nutrition*, *119*(10), 1087–1101. https://doi.org/***10.1017/S0007114518000697***

111. Sampath, S., Mahapatra, S. C., Padhi, M. M., Sharma, R., & Talwar, A. (2015). Holy basil (Ocimum sanctum Linn.) leaf extract enhances specific cognitive parameters in healthy adult volunteers: A placebo controlled study. *Indian Journal of Physiology and Pharmacology*, *59*(1), 69–77. ***https://pubmed.ncbi.nlm.nih.gov/26571987/***

112. Sarris, J., Logan, A. C., Akbaraly, T. N., Amminger, G. P., Balanzá-Martínez, V., Freeman, M. P., Hibbeln, J., Matsuoka, Y., Mischoulon, D., Mizoue, T., Nanri, A., Nishi, D., Ramsey, D., Rucklidge, J. J., Sanchez-Villegas, A., Scholey, A., Su, K.-P., & Jacka, F. N. (2015). Nutritional medicine as mainstream in psychiatry. *The Lancet Psychiatry*, *2*(3), 271–274. https://doi.org/***10.1016/s2215-0366(14)00051-0***

113. Scholey, A., Gibbs, A., Neale, C., Perry, N., Ossoukhova, A., Bilog, V., Kras, M., Scholz, C., Sass, M., & Buchwald-Werner, S. (2014). Anti-Stress Effects of Lemon Balm-Containing Foods. *Nutrients*, *6*(11), 4805–4821. https://doi.org/***10.3390/nu6114805***

114. Schütz, K., Sass, M., de With, A., Graubaum, H.-J., & Grünwald, J. (2010). Immune-modulating efficacy of a polyphenol-rich beverage on symptoms associated with the common cold: a double-blind, randomised, placebo-controlled, multi-centric clinical study. *The British Journal of Nutrition*, *104*(8), 1156–1164. https://doi.org/***10.1017/S0007114510002047***

115. Sgarbanti, R., Amatore, D., Celestino, I., Marcocci, M. E., Fraternale, A., Ciriolo, M. R., Magnani, M., Saladino, R., Garaci, E., Palamara, A. T., & Nencioni, L. (2014). Intracellular Redox State as Target for Anti-Influenza Therapy: Are Antioxidants Always Effective? *Current Topics in Medicinal Chemistry*, *14*(22), 2529–2541. https://doi.org/**10.2174/1568026614666141203125211**

116. Shankar, A. H., & Prasad, A. S. (1998). Zinc and immune function: the biological basis of altered resistance to infection. *The American Journal of Clinical Nutrition*, *68*(2), 447S463S. https://doi.org/**10.1093/ajcn/68.2.447s**

117. Singh, A. V. (2003). Sulforaphane induces caspase-mediated apoptosis in cultured PC-3 human prostate cancer cells and retards growth of PC-3 xenografts in vivo. *Carcinogenesis*, *25*(1), 83–90. https://doi.org/**10.1093/carcin/bgg178**

118. Somerville, V. S., Braakhuis, A. J., & Hopkins, W. G. (2016). Effect of Flavonoids on Upper Respiratory Tract Infections and Immune Function: A Systematic Review and Meta-Analysis. *Advances in Nutrition*, *7*(3), 488–497. https://doi.org/**10.3945/an.115.010538**

119. Spedding, S. (2014). Vitamin D and Depression: A Systematic Review and Meta-Analysis Comparing Studies with and without Biological Flaws. *Nutrients*, *6*(4), 1501–1518. https://doi.org/**10.3390/nu6041501**

120. Stephens, W. (2019). *Probiotics May Benefit Patients With Parkinson Disease.* AJMC. ***https://www.ajmc.com/view/probiotics-may-benefit-patients-with-parkinson-disease***

121. Stoodley, I., Garg, M., Scott, H., Macdonald-Wicks, L., Berthon, B., & Wood, L. (2019). Higher Omega-3 Index Is Associated with Better Asthma Control and Lower Medication Dose: A Cross-Sectional Study. *Nutrients*, *12*(1), 74. https://doi.org/**10.3390/nu12010074**

122. Su, K.-P., Matsuoka, Y., & Pae, C.-U. (2015). Omega-3 Polyunsaturated Fatty Acids in Prevention of Mood and Anxiety Disorders. *Clinical Psychopharmacology and Neuroscience*, *13*(2), 129–137. https://doi.org/**10.9758/cpn.2015.13.2.129**

123. Takada, M., Nishida, K., Kataoka-Kato, A., Gondo, Y., Ishikawa, H., Suda, K., Kawai, M., Hoshi, R., Watanabe, O., Igarashi, T., Kuwano, Y., Miyazaki, K., & Rokutan, K. (2016). Probiotic Lactobacillus casei strain Shirota relieves stress-associated symptoms by modulating the gut–brain interaction in human and animal models. *Neurogastroenterology & Motility*, *28*(7), 1027–1036. https://doi.org/**10.1111/nmo.12804**

124. Tillisch, K., Labus, J., Kilpatrick, L., Jiang, Z., Stains, J., Ebrat, B., Guyonnet, D., Legrain–Raspaud, S., Trotin, B., Naliboff, B., & Mayer, E. A. (2013). Consumption of Fermented Milk Product With Probiotic Modulates Brain Activity. *Gastroenterology*, *144*(7), 1394-1401.e4. https://doi.org/**10.1053/j.gastro.2013.02.043**

125. Vighi, G., Marcucci, F., Sensi, L., Di Cara, G., & Frati, F. (2008). Allergy and the gastrointestinal system. *Clinical & Experimental Immunology*, *153*, 3–6. https://doi.org/**10.1111/j.1365-2249.2008.03713.x**

126.   Wang, Y., Li, X., Ge, T., Xiao, Y., Liao, Y., Cui, Y., Zhang, Y., Ho, W., Yu, G., & Zhang, T. (2016). Probiotics for prevention and treatment of respiratory tract infections in children. *Medicine*, *95*(31), e4509. https://doi.org/**10.1097/md.0000000000004509**

127. Webb, D. (2016a). *Health at Every Size: A Dietary Approach that Focuses on Healthful Lifestyle Behaviors — Not Weight Loss - Today's Dietitian Magazine*. Todaysdietitian.com. **https://www.todaysdietitian.com/newarchives/0116p26.shtml**

128.   Webb, D. (2016b). *Herbs and Spices: Holiday Spices - Today's Dietitian Magazine*. Www.todaysdietitian.com. **https://www.todaysdietitian.com/newarchives/1116p14.shtml**

129.   Wright, K. C. (2019, July). *Clinical Nutrition: Beyond Food and Mood - Today's Dietitian Magazine*. Www.todaysdietitian.com. **https://www.todaysdietitian.com/newarchives/0719p10.shtml**

130.   Wright, M. L., Fournier, C., Houser, M. C., Tansey, M., Glass, J., & Hertzberg, V. S. (2018). Potential Role of the Gut Microbiome in ALS: A Systematic Review. *Biological Research for Nursing*, *20*(5), 513–521. https://doi.org/**10.1177/1099800418784202**

131. Wu, L., Wang, Z., Zhu, J., Murad, A. L., Prokop, L. J., & Murad, M. H. (2015). Nut consumption and risk of cancer and type 2 diabetes: a systematic review and meta-analysis. *Nutrition Reviews*, *73*(7), 409–425. https://doi.org/**10.1093/nutrit/nuv006**

132.   Xiao, J., Wang, T., Xu, Y., Gu, X., Li, D., Niu, K., Wang, T., Zhao, J., Zhou, R., & Wang, H.-L. (2020). Long-term probiotic intervention mitigates memory dysfunction through a novel H3K27me3-based mechanism in lead-exposed rats. *Translational Psychiatry*, *10*(1), 25. https://doi.org/**10.1038/s41398-020-0719-8**

133.   Zandi, P. P. (2004). Reduced Risk of Alzheimer Disease in Users of Antioxidant Vitamin Supplements. *Archives of Neurology*, *61*(1), 82. https://doi.org/**10.1001/archneur.61.1.82**

About the Expert

Lacy Ngo, MS, RDN, is a registered dietitian with a Master's of Science in Human Nutrition. She is an expert in health, wellness, and weight loss and has extensive professional and personal health transformation experience. Ngo lost 50 pounds and has since helped her clients transform their health by sharing her best health transformation strategies. Ngo is the author of several books and has been quoted and featured in media outlets like Parade, Eat This, Not That!, The Healthy, CN2 News, and Authority Magazine. Ngo also finished 5th in her group in the Ms. Health and Fitness Competition.

HowExpert publishes 'how to' guides by everyday experts. Visit HowExpert.com to learn more.

Recommended Resources

- HowExpert.com – Quick 'How To' Guides on All Topics from A to Z by Everyday Experts.
- HowExpert.com/free – Free HowExpert Email Newsletter.
- HowExpert.com/books – HowExpert Books
- HowExpert.com/courses – HowExpert Courses
- HowExpert.com/clothing – HowExpert Clothing
- HowExpert.com/membership – HowExpert Membership Site
- HowExpert.com/affiliates – HowExpert Affiliate Program
- HowExpert.com/jobs – HowExpert Jobs
- HowExpert.com/writers – Write About Your #1 Passion/Knowledge/Expertise & Become a HowExpert Author.
- HowExpert.com/resources – Additional HowExpert Recommended Resources
- YouTube.com/HowExpert – Subscribe to HowExpert YouTube.
- Instagram.com/HowExpert – Follow HowExpert on Instagram.
- Facebook.com/HowExpert – Follow HowExpert on Facebook.
- TikTok.com/@HowExpert – Follow HowExpert on TikTok.

Printed in Great Britain
by Amazon

15983289R00109